How to Display Data

How to Display Data

Jenny V. Freeman

School of Health and Related Research
University of Sheffield
Sheffield, UK

Stephen J. Walters

School of Health and Related Research
University of Sheffield
Sheffield, UK

Michael J. Campbell

School of Health and Related Research
University of Sheffield
Sheffield, UK

BMJ|Books

Blackwell
Publishing

Blackwell Publishing, Inc., 350 Main Street, Malden, Massachusetts 02148-5020, USA
Blackwell Publishing Ltd, 9600 Garsington Road, Oxford OX4 2DQ, UK
Blackwell Publishing Asia Pty Ltd, 550 Swanston Street, Carlton, Victoria 3053, Australia

First published 2008

1 2008

Library of Congress Cataloging-in-Publication Data
Freeman, Jenny.
How to display data / Jenny Freeman, Stephen J. Walters, Michael J. Campbell.
    p. ; cm.
  ISBN 978-1-4051-3974-8 (pbk. : alk. paper)
  1. Medical writing. 2. Medical statistics. 3. Medicine–Research–Statistical methods.
I. Walters, Stephen John. II. Campbell, Michael J., PhD. III. Title. [DNLM: 1. Research Design. 2. Data Display. 3. Data Interpretation, Statistical. 4. Statistics. W 20.5 F869h 2007]
  R119.F76 2007
  610.72′7–dc22

                                                                        2007032641

ISBN: 978-1-4051-3974-8

A catalogue record for this title is available from the British Library

Set by Charon Tec Ltd (A Macmillan Company), Chennai, India
Printed and bound in Singapore by Utopia Press Pte Ltd

Commissioning Editor: Mary Banks
Editorial Assistant: Victoria Pittman
Development Editor: Simone Dudziak
Production Controller: Rachel Edwards

For further information on Blackwell Publishing, visit our website:
http://www.blackwellpublishing.com

Contents

Preface

The best method to convey a message from a piece of research in health is via a figure. The best advice that a statistician can give a researcher is to first plot the data. Despite this, conventional statistics textbooks give only brief details on how to draw figures and display data. The purpose of this book is to give advice on the best methods to display data which have arisen from a variety of different sources. We have tried to make the book concise and easy to read. By displaying data badly one can very easily give misleading messages (or hide inconvenient truths) and we try to highlight how consumers of data have to be aware of these problems. We have also included advice on displaying data for posters and talks.

Researchers who want to display the results of their studies in figures or tables particularly for publication in a journal will find this book useful. Readers of the research literature, who wish to critically appraise a piece of work will find useful tips on interpreting figures that they encounter. People who have to deliver a talk or a conference presentation should also find good advice on displaying their results.

We would like to thank Mary Banks and Simone Dudziak from Blackwell for their patience and advice.

Jenny V. Freeman
Stephen J. Walters
Michael J. Campbell
Medical Statistics Group, ScHARR, Sheffield
June 2007

Chapter 1 **Introduction to data display**

1.1 Introduction

This book has arisen from our extensive experience as researchers and teachers of medical statistics. We have frequently been appalled by the poor quality of data display even in major medical journals. While there is already a wealth of information about how to display data, it is scattered across many sources. Our purpose in writing this book is to bring together this information into a single volume and provide clear accessible advice for both researchers, and students alike.

Well-displayed data can clearly illuminate and enhance the interpretation of a study, while badly laid out data and results can obscure the message or at worst seriously mislead. Although the appropriate display of data in tables and graphs is an essential part of any report, paper or presentation, little space is devoted to it in the majority of textbooks. The purpose of this book is to address this deficit and give clear guidelines on appropriate methods for displaying quantitative information, using both graphs and tables.

There are many different types of graph and table available for displaying data; their purposes will be outlined in subsequent chapters. This chapter will outline the reasons why it is important to get display right, good principles to adhere to when displaying data and the types of data that will be covered in the rest of the book. The second chapter will cover some of the many ways in which the display of information can be badly done and the following chapters will then unpick these, and give clear guidance on how to do it well.

1.2 Types of data

To display data appropriately, one must first understand what types of data there are, as this determines the best method of displaying them. Figure 1.1 shows a basic hierarchy of data types, although there are others. Data are either *categorical* or *quantitative*. Data are described as categorical when they can

1

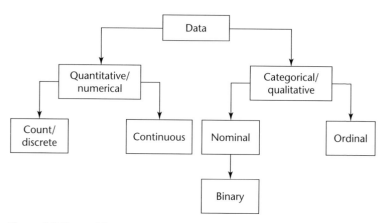

Figure 1.1 Types of data.

be categorised into distinct groups, such as ethnic group or disease severity. Although categorical data may be coded numerically, for example gender may be coded 1 for male and 2 for female, these codes have no intrinsic numerical value; it would be nonsense to calculate an average gender. Categorical data can be divided into either *nominal* or *ordinal*. Nominal data have no natural ordering and examples include eye colour, marital status and area of residence. *Binary* data is a special subcategory of nominal data, where there are only two possible values, for example male/female, yes/no, dead/alive. Ordinal data occurs when there can be said to be a natural ordering of the data values, such as better/same/worse, grades of breast cancer and social class.

Quantitative data can be either counted or continuous. *Count* data are also known as discrete data and, as the name implies, occur when the data can be counted, such as the number of children in a family or the number of visits to a GP in a year. Count data are similar to categorical data as they can only take discrete whole numbers. *Continuous* data are data that can be measured and they can take any value on the scale on which they are measured; they are limited only by the scale of measurement and examples include height, weight and blood pressure.

1.3 Where to start?

When displaying information visually, there are three questions one will find useful to ask as a starting point (Box 1.1). Firstly and most importantly, it is vital to have a clear idea about what is to be displayed; for example, is it important to demonstrate that two sets of data have different distributions or

> **Box 1.1** Useful questions to ask when considering how to display information
>
> • What do you want to show?
> • What methods are available for this?
> • Is the method chosen the best? Would another have been better?

that they have different mean values? Having decided what the main message is, the next step is to examine the methods available and to select an appropriate one. Finally, once the chart or table has been constructed, it is worth reflecting upon whether what has been produced truly reflects the intended message. If not, then refine the display until satisfied; for example if a chart has been used would a table have been better or vice versa? This book will help you answer these questions and provide you with the means to best display your data.

1.4 Recommendations for the presentation of numbers

When summarising categorical data, both frequencies and percentages can be used. However, if percentages are reported, it is important that the denominator (i.e. total number of observations) is given. To summarise continuous numerical data, one should use the mean and standard deviation, or if the data have a skewed distribution use the median and range or interquartile range. However, for all of these calculated quantities it is important to state the total number of observations on which they are based.

In the majority of cases it is reasonable to treat count data, such as number of children in a family or number of visits to the GP in a year, as if they were continuous, at least as far as the statistical analysis goes. Ideally there should be a large number of different possible values, but in practice this is not always necessary. However, where ordered categories are numbered, such as stage of disease or social class, the temptation to treat these numbers as statistically meaningful must be resisted. For example, it is not sensible to calculate the average social class of a sample or stage of cancer for a group of patients, and in such cases the data should be treated in statistical analyses as if they are ordered categories.[1]

Numerical precision should be consistent throughout and summary statistics such as means and standard deviations should not have more than one extra decimal place (or significant digit) compared to the raw data. Spurious precision should be avoided although when certain measures are to be used for further calculations or when presenting the results of analyses, greater precision may sometimes be appropriate.[2]

1.5 Recommendations for presenting data and results in tables

There are a few basic rules of good presentation, both within the text of a document or presentation, and within tables, as outlined in Box 1.2. Tufte, in 1983, outlined a fundamental principle: always try to get as much information into a figure consistent with legibility. In other words, one should maximise the ratio of the amount of information given to the amount of ink used.[3] Tables, including column and row headings, should be clearly labelled and a brief summary of the contents of a table should always be given in words, either as part of the title or in the main body of the text.

Box 1.2 Recommendations when presenting data and results in tables

- The amount of information should be maximised for the minimum amount of ink.
- Numerical precision should be consistent throughout a paper or presentation, as far as possible.
- Avoid spurious accuracy. Numbers should be rounded to two effective digits.
- Quantitative data should be summarised using either the mean and standard deviation (for symmetrically distributed data) or the median and interquartile range or range (for skewed data). The number of observations on which these summary measures are based should be included.
- Categorical data should be summarised as frequencies and percentages. As with quantitative data, the number of observations should be included.
- Each table should have a title explaining what is being displayed and columns and rows should be clearly labelled.
- Solid lines in tables should be kept to a minimum.
- Where variables have no natural ordering, rows and columns should be ordered by size.

Solid lines should not be used in a table except to separate labels and summary measures from the main body of the data. However, their use should be kept to a minimum, particularly vertical gridlines, as they can interrupt eye movements, and thus the flow of information. White space can be used to separate data, such as different variables, from each other.[4]

The information in tables is easier to comprehend if the columns (rather than the rows) contain similar information, such as means or standard deviations, as it is easier to scan down a column than across a row.[4] However, it is not always easy to do this, particularly when the information for several variables is contained in the same table and comparisons are to be made between different groups. This will be covered in more detail in Chapter 6. In addition, where there is no natural ordering of the rows (or indeed columns), they should be ordered by size (category with the highest frequency first, lowest frequency last) as this helps the reader to scan for patterns and exceptions in the data.[4] Table 1.1a shows the frequency distribution for marital status for 226 patients with leg ulcers who were recruited to a study to assess the effectiveness of specialist leg ulcers clinics compared to usual care.[5] The categories in this table are ordered alphabetically, whereas in Table 1.1b the marital status categories are ordered by frequency making it much easier to interpret than Table 1.1a.

Table 1.1 Marital status of 226 patients with leg ulcer recruited to a study to assess the effectiveness of specialist leg ulcer clinics using 4-layer compression bandaging compared to usual care[5]

	Frequency	Percent
(a) Unordered rows		
Divorced/separated	11	4.9
Married	104	46.0
Single	25	11.1
Widowed	86	38.1
Total	226	100.0
(b) Ordered rows		
Married	104	46.0
Widowed	86	38.1
Single	25	11.1
Divorced/separated	11	4.9
Total	226	100.0

1.6 Recommendations for construction of graphs

Box 1.3 outlines some basic recommendations for the construction and use of figures to display data. As with tables, a fundamental principle is that graphs should maximise the amount of information presented for the minimum amount of ink used.[3] Good graphs have the following four features in common: clarity of message, simplicity of design, clarity of text, and integrity of intention and action.[6] A graph should have a title explaining what is displayed and axes should be clearly labelled; if it is not immediately

Box 1.3 Guidelines for constructing graphs

• The amount of information should be maximised for the minimum amount of ink.
• Each graph should have a title explaining what is being displayed.
• Axes should be clearly labelled.
• Gridlines should be kept to a minimum.
• Avoid three-dimensional graphs as these can be difficult to read.
• The number of observations should be included.

obvious how many individuals the graph is based upon, this should also be stated. Gridlines should be kept to a minimum as they act as a distraction and can interrupt the flow of information. When using graphs for presentation purposes care must be taken to ensure that they are not misleading; an excellent exposition of the ways in which graphs can be used to mislead can be found in Huff.[7] Figure 1.2 shows a bar chart of the marital status data from Table 1.1 displayed using these principles. It includes a clear title (with the sample size), labelled axes, no gridlines and the marital status categories are ordered by their frequency.

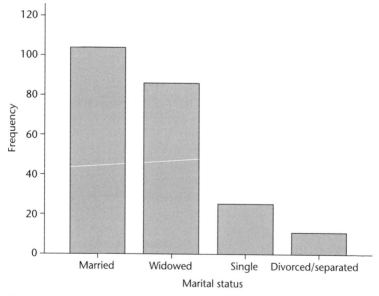

Figure 1.2 Bar chart of marital status for 226 patients recruited to the leg ulcer Study.[5]

1.7 Table or graph?

A fundamental point to consider is whether to use a table or graph (see Box 1.4). We define a table as a display of numbers in a rectangular grid, and a graph or chart as a picture in which the numbers are represented by points or lines. Plotting data is a useful first stage to any analysis and will show extreme observations together with any discernible patterns. In addition the relative sizes of categories are easier to see in a diagram (bar chart or pie chart) than in a table. Graphs are useful as they can be assimilated quickly, and are particularly helpful when presenting information to an audience. Tables can be useful for displaying information about many variables at once, while graphs can be useful for showing multiple observations on groups or individuals. Although there are no hard and fast rules about when to use a graph and when to use a table, in the context of a report or a paper it is often best to use tables so that the reader can scrutinise the numbers directly. Thus, for a talk or presentation, Figure 1.2 would be a good method of displaying the data. However, for a printed report or paper, Table 1.1b conveys the data more accurately and succinctly.

Box 1.4 Graph or table	
Graph	Table
Usually better in presentations	Often better in papers
Can often show all the data	Usually can only show summaries
Usually show only a few variables	Better for multiple variables

1.8 Software

No single package can draw all the graphs necessary for displaying data. Simple graphs can be drawn in *Microsoft Excel*. However, you should be aware that some of the default settings are not ideal (see Chapter 2). For more complex graphs, any of the major statistical packages – *STATA*, *SPSS* or *SAS* – are useful. *S-Plus* is particularly good for superimposing several graphs into a single figure. In drawing the graphs for this book a variety of packages were used, although many were drawn in the specialist package Sigmaplot (Systat Software Inc 24, Vista Centre, 50, Salisbury Road, Hounslow, TW4 6JQ, London). Packages change regularly so we have not given explicit instructions on how to draw individual graphs in particular packages. The book simply outlines good practice for displaying data.

Summary

- The purpose of any attempt to present data and results, either in a presentation or on paper is to communicate with an audience.
- In the following chapters key methods using both graphs and tables will be outlined so that by the end of this book you should have the skills and knowledge to display your data appropriately.
- In addition, you will be able to distinguish between bad graphs and good graphs and know how to transform the former into the latter and you should be able to distinguish between a bad table and a good table and be able to transform the former into the latter.
- A variety of software packages is available for drawing graphs. In order to draw all of the graphs outlined in this book you will need to use several packages.

References

1 Freeman JV, Walters SJ. Examining relationships in quantitative data (inferential statistics). In: Gerrish K, Lacey A, editors. *The research process in nursing*, 5th ed. Oxford: Blackwell; 2006, pp. 454–74.

2 Altman DG, Bland JM. Presentation of numerical data. *British Medical Journal* 1996;**312**:572.

3 Tufte ER. *The visual display of quantitative information.* Cheshire, Connecticut: Graphics Press; 1983.

4 Ehrenberg ASC. *A primer in data reduction.* Chichester: John Wiley & Sons; 2000.

5 Morrell CJ, Walters SJ, Dixon S, Collins K, Brereton LML, Peters J, et al. Cost effectiveness of community leg ulcer clinic: randomised controlled trial. *British Medical Journal* 1998;**316**:1487–91.

6 Bigwood S, Spore M. *Presenting numbers, tables and charts.* Oxford: Oxford University Press; 2003.

7 Huff D. *How to lie with statistics.* London: Penguin Books; 1991.

Chapter 2 **How to display data badly**

2.1 Introduction

There are a great many ways in which data can be badly displayed and this chapter outlines some of the more common errors. This topic is covered in greater depth by Huff in his classic text 'How to lie with Statistics', in which he lays out the numerous ways in which poorly displayed data can be used to mislead.[1] A further useful reference is Wainer.[2]

2.2 Amount of information

One of the easiest ways to display data badly is to display as little information as possible. This includes not labelling axes and titles adequately, and not giving units. In addition, information that is displayed can be obscured by including unnecessary and distracting details.

Consider the following simple data set resulting from a survey of students (Table 2.1).

Table 2.1 Height of 10 students (in centimetres)

Men	Women
175	179
180	160
171	165
175	170
185	174

A common way to display these data badly is to present the means for each group and their associated standard errors using a bar chart with error bars, so called 'dynamite plunger plots' as shown in Figure 2.1.

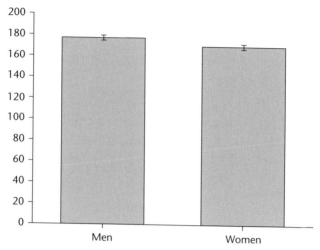

Figure 2.1 Mean and standard error bars of data in Table 2.1 displayed using a bar chart.

This chart violates many of the recommendations of Chapter 1 and yet is commonplace. While only four pieces of information are displayed (group means and their standard errors) much ink is wasted drawing the bars. The scale begins at the origin, so that the variability of the data is compressed into a small area. The Y-axis is not clearly labelled as there is no indication of the scale and no information about the number of observations in each group. Most importantly for these data, the raw data are hidden behind a summary statistic. It may be that the purpose of displaying these data is to compare the group means, in which case a better way would be simply to report these statistics in the text. However, if the reason for displaying data such as these is to compare the spread of values in the two groups, the standard errors for the individual means are of little use and you are better just showing the actual data, using a dot plot as described in Chapter 4.

It is possible to become even more obscure by using a three-dimensional chart and vertical axis that does not start at zero as shown in Figure 2.2.

We have now succeeded in showing only two pieces of information (the mean values of height for men and women) and also managed to obscure them by gratuitously making the chart three dimensional. Furthermore, the difference in mean height between the male and female students has been exaggerated by making the Y-axis start at 164 cm.

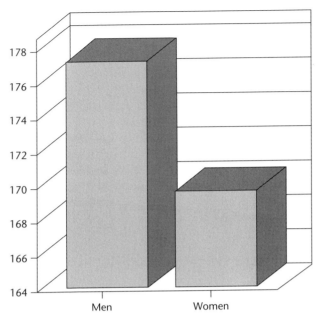

Figure 2.2 Three-dimensional bar chart of data in Table 2.1.

2.3 Suppress the origin or change the baseline

A frequent means of exaggerating trends over time is to suppress the origin. This type of error creates the 'gee-whiz' graph for showing trends.[1] Table 2.2 contains the age-standardised death rates for women, in England and Wales, from lung cancer for the years 1998–2004.[3] By starting the Y-axis at 282 deaths per million, a relatively small decrease from 291 to 284 deaths per million looks very dramatic. The type of graph displayed in Figure 2.3 is common and shows an apparently large change, whereas the actual decrease represents a fall of about 2.4% over a 7-year period.

Table 2.2 Age-standardised death rates from lung cancer (per million) for women in England and Wales for the years 1998–2004, using the European Standard Population[3]

Year	1998	1999	2000	2001	2002	2003	2004
Death rate	291	289	285	283	284	285	284

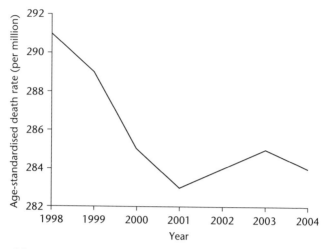

Figure 2.3 Age-standardised death rates from lung cancer (per million) for women in England and Wales for the years 1998–2004, using the European Standard Population.[3]

The baseline that groups are compared to can be further obscured in other less deliberate ways than by simply changing the origin. Figure 2.4 shows the age-standardised death rates from different causes in the UK from 1996 to 2005, for women. The death rates from the different causes have been stacked on top of each other for each year. In practice only the deaths from COPD and the total deaths from all seven causes can be compared simply over time. This is because the baseline for the other causes changes with time. It is difficult to decide for the majority of other causes whether there are any changes over time (with the possible exception of cerebrovascular disease and heart disease). These data might be more usefully displayed by presenting the different rates as different lines, with the same Y-axis, as shown in Figure 2.5.

2.4 Don't order the data by value

For categorical data with no intrinsic order to the categories, a particularly good way to obscure any patterns in the data is to order the categories arbitrarily, for example alphabetically. Figure 2.6 shows the population size, in 2004, for 20 European countries.[4] The countries are displayed in alphabetical order. In this case, while the most populous country, Germany, can be readily seen, for countries of similar sizes, such as France, Italy and the

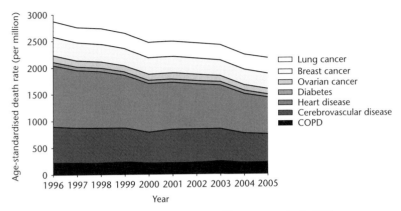

Figure 2.4 Age-standardised death rates from different causes in the UK by year (1996–2005), for women; death rates stacked on top of each other cumulatively.[3]

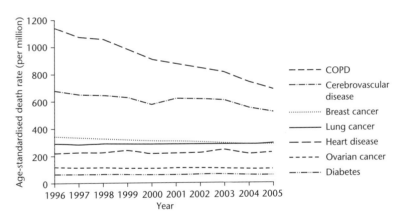

Figure 2.5 Age-standardised death rates from different causes in the UK by year (1996–2005), for women; death rates plotted individually.[3]

UK, it is not immediately obvious which has the largest population. It would be better to order these data by size as shown in Figure 2.7, where it can be easily seen that of the three countries mentioned above, Italy has the smallest population, France the largest and the UK lies between these two.[5] It then becomes much clearer how each country relates to the others in Europe with respect to population size.

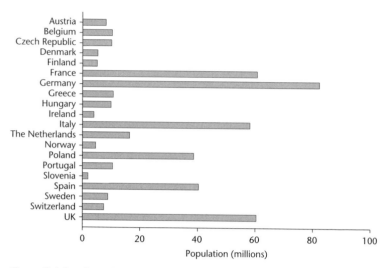

Figure 2.6 Population (in millions), in 2004, for 20 European countries ordered by alphabetically.[4]

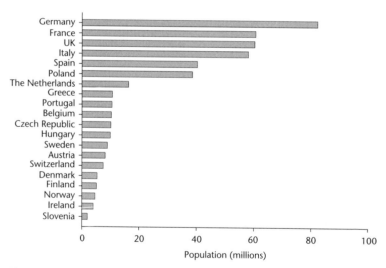

Figure 2.7 Population (in millions), in 2004, for 20 European countries ordered by size.[4]

2.5 Use images to show linear contrasts

Figure 2.8 shows a chart contrasting the average earnings of UK doctors and nurses, by using symbols, money bags in this case, to represent the actual

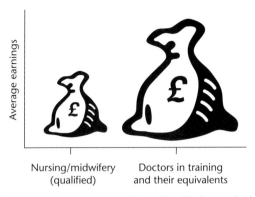

Figure 2.8 UK average earnings (in £s), in 2004, of qualified nurses/midwives compared to doctors in training and their equivalents.[6]

data values.[6] This type of chart is a particular favourite of newspapers. Rather than displaying the actual numbers, solid figures or images are used instead. While this again produces the 'gee-whiz' graph it should be discouraged for scientific work because the eye automatically contrasts areas rather than the heights of the symbols, and area increases as the *square* of height and thus makes the contrast more impressive. These figures are best displayed by giving the actual numbers.

Summary

In order to display data badly you need to:
• Display as little information as you can.
• Obscure what information you do show with distracting additions (also known as chart junk).
• Use a poor scale or suppress the origin.
• Use pseudo-three-dimensional charts.
• Use colour or pattern gratuitously.
• Use symbols or images of different sizes to represent the frequencies for different groups.

References

1 Huff D. *How to lie with statistics*. London: Penguin Books; 1991.
2 Wainer H. How to display data badly. *The American Statistician* 1984;**38**:137–47.

3 *Mortaility statistics: cause.* Report No.: 32. London: Office for National Statistics; 2006.

4 Schott B. *Schott's almanac.* London: Bloomsbury; 2006.

5 Ehrenberg ASC. *A primer in data reduction.* Chichester: John Wiley & Sons; 2000.

6 *NHS staff earnings survey: August 2004.* Leeds: NHS Health and Social Care Information Centre; 2005.

Chapter 3 **Displaying univariate categorical data**

3.1 Describing categorical data

This chapter will concentrate on appropriate ways of displaying categorical data; that is data that can be categorised into groups, such as blood group or disease severity.

An initial step when describing categorical data is to count the number of observations in each category and express them as percentages of the total sample size. For example, Table 3.1 contains categorical data from a self-completed postal questionnaire survey of new mothers approximately 8 weeks post delivery.[1] One of the questions the mothers were asked was 'What kind of delivery did you have?' To display categorical data such as these we can use either pie charts or bar charts. Note that these categories are ordered by size: it is immediately obvious which are the most/least frequent categories.

Table 3.1 Self-reported type of delivery for new mothers ($n = 3221$)[1]

What kind of delivery?	Number in each category (%)	
Normal vaginal delivery	2221	(69.0)
Emergency caesarean section (once labour had started)	434	(13.5)
Planned caesarean section	251	(7.8)
Ventouse (vacuum extractor)	210	(6.5)
Forceps delivery	89	(2.7)
Vaginal breech delivery	16	(0.5)
Total	3221	(100.0)

3.2 Pie charts

Figure 3.1 displays the data in Table 3.1 as a pie chart (so-called because it resembles a pie cut into pieces for serving). Each segment in the pie chart

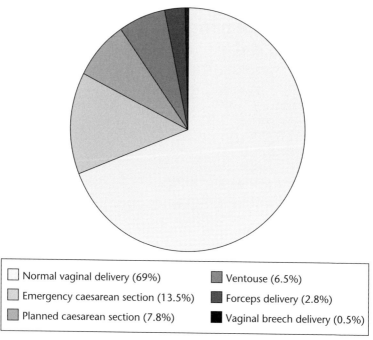

Figure 3.1 Pie chart of self-reported type of delivery for all new mothers, using shading to distinguish between different categories (n = 3221).[1]

represents an individual category. The area displayed for each category is proportional to the number in that category. A pie chart is constructed by dividing a circle into sectors, with each sector (or segment) representing a different category. The angle of each segment is proportional to the relative frequency for that segment. This angle is calculated by multiplying the proportion in each category by 360 (as there are 360 degrees in a circle) to give the corresponding angle in degrees. This is demonstrated in Table 3.2. If you regard the chart as a clock then it is good practice to always start at 12 o'clock and proceed in a clockwise direction around the circle. Where there is no natural ordering to the categories it can be helpful to order them by size,[2] as this can help you to pick out any patterns or compare the relative frequencies across groups. As it can be difficult to discern immediately the numbers represented in each of the categories it is good practice to include the number of observations on which the chart is based, together with the percentages in each category.

While it is possible to use different colours to distinguish between the different groups, colour should be employed with caution. A photocopy of the chart may have different colours appearing the same which makes it hard to

Table 3.2 Calculations for a pie chart of type of delivery for new mothers[1]

What kind of delivery?	Proportion in category (P)	Angle of the segment (P*360)
Normal vaginal delivery	0.690	248.4
Emergency caesarean section (once labour had started)	0.135	48.6
Planned caesarean section	0.078	28.1
Ventouse (vacuum extractor)	0.065	23.4
Forceps delivery	0.027	9.7
Vaginal breech delivery	0.005	1.8
Total	1.000	360

distinguish between the categories. An alternative would be to use different patterns, but again this should be done carefully as different patterns can have the effect of making the chart look very busy (as shown in Figure 3.2). It is safest to use different shades of the same colour to represent different groups, as has been done in Figure 3.1.

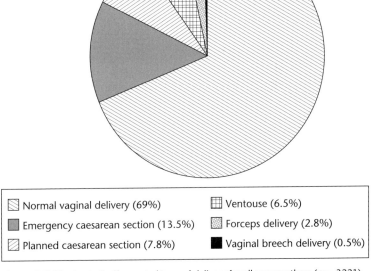

Normal vaginal delivery (69%)   Ventouse (6.5%)

Emergency caesarean section (13.5%)   Forceps delivery (2.8%)

Planned caesarean section (7.8%)   Vaginal breech delivery (0.5%)

Figure 3.2 Pie chart of self-reported type of delivery for all new mothers (n = 3221), using pattern to distinguish between different categories.[1]

Generally pie charts are to be avoided, as they can be difficult to interpret particularly when the number of categories is greater than five. Small proportions can be very hard to discern, as is the case for vaginal breech delivery here. In addition, unless the percentages in each of the individual categories are given as numbers it can be much more difficult to estimate them from a pie chart than from a bar chart, as described in the next section.

3.3 Bar charts

A better way of displaying categorical data than a pie chart is to use a bar chart, such as Figure 3.3. The categories for the different methods of delivery are listed along the horizontal axis, while the number in each category is on the vertical axis. As with pie charts the area displayed for each category should be proportional to the number in that category. Although the vertical scale for this graph is the frequency, this could easily be rescaled to percentages. There are advantages to both types of scale and the shape of the resultant

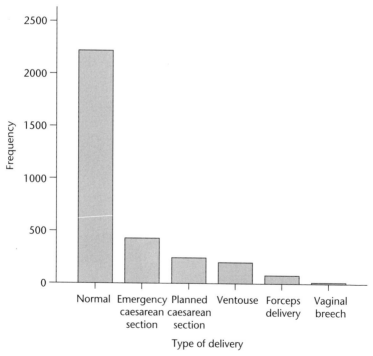

Figure 3.3 Bar chart of self-reported type of delivery for all new mothers ($n = 3221$).[1]

chart will not be affected by the choice of scale. The advantage of using the frequencies is that the numbers in each category on the horizontal (X) axis can be readily seen. Using the percentage scale the percentages in each category can be easily discerned. Use of the percentage scale facilitates the comparison of groups, as in Figure 3.5. Where there is no natural ordering to the categories it can again be helpful to order them by size.

3.4 Two- or three-dimensional charts?

It is common practice to display data such as that in Table 3.1 as a three-dimensional bar chart or pie chart (Figure 3.4). However, this should *never* be done as they are especially difficult to read and interpret as discussed in Chapter 2. The area displayed should be proportional to the relative frequencies for each group. However, when the charts are displayed as three dimensional this relationship is lost as what is displayed becomes a volume. Only the front face is proportional to the numbers in the categories and so only these should be displayed, as in Figures 3.1–3.3. In particular, categories with only a few individuals are given undue weight in three-dimensional charts as the top face is much more prominent. Consider for example the vaginal breech births category in Figure 3.3. There are only 16

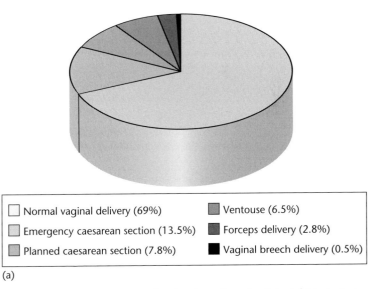

Normal vaginal delivery (69%)	Ventouse (6.5%)
Emergency caesarean section (13.5%)	Forceps delivery (2.8%)
Planned caesarean section (7.8%)	Vaginal breech delivery (0.5%)

(a)

Figure 3.4 Data for all women displayed as three-dimensional charts:[1] (a) pie chart and (b) bar chart (see over).

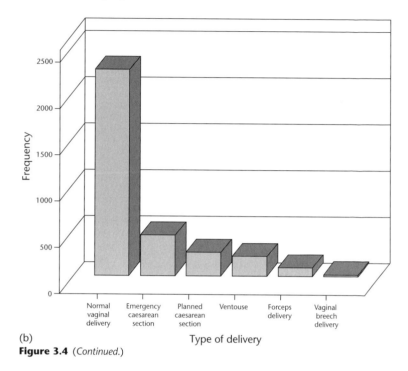

(b)

Figure 3.4 (*Continued.*)

individuals in this category compared to 2221 in the normal delivery category and so vaginal breech births comprise <1% of births. However this is not the impression given in Figure 3.4. Above all else, a graph should be simple and accurately reflect the data so that the reader can easily understand the information being conveyed. Neither Figure 3.4 nor b do this and should not be used. A final point about three-dimensional bar charts is that it can be hard to read the scale, particularly for those bars furthest away from the scale markers, as it is not clear whether the scale should be read from the left or from the back.

While Figures 3.1 and 3.3 are less visually exciting than Figure 3.4a and b they are much clearer and less ambiguous and more accurately reflect the data.

3.5 Clustered bar charts

The data in Table 3.1 can be further classified into whether or not the baby is the first (primiparous) or subsequent child (multiparous) (Table 3.3). It now becomes impossible to present the data as a single pie chart or bar

Table 3.3 Self-reported type of delivery for new mothers ($n = 3221$)[1]

What kind of delivery?	Primiparous (%)	Multiparous (%)
Normal vaginal delivery	857 (58.1)	1364 (78.2)
Emergency caesarean section (once labour had started)	302 (20.5)	132 (7.6)
Planned caesarean section	72 (4.9)	179 (10.3)
Ventouse (vacuum extractor)	162 (11.0)	48 (2.8)
Forceps delivery	76 (5.1)	13 (0.7)
Vaginal breech delivery	7 (0.5)	9 (0.5)
Total	1476 (100.0)	1745 (100.0)

chart. These data are categorised in two ways, by type of delivery and parity, enabling the distribution of delivery type to be compared between those women who had no previous children and those who had at least one. Table 3.3 is an example of a 6 × 2 *contingency table* with 6 rows (representing type of delivery) and 2 columns (representing parity) and it is said to have 12 cells (6 × 2). More generally, a contingency table with *r* rows and *c* columns is known as an *r* by *c* contingency table and has *r* × *c* cells. Type of delivery is said to have been *cross-tabulated* with parity.

The data could be presented as two separate pie charts or bar charts side by side but it is preferable to present the data in one graph with the same scales and axes to make the visual comparisons easier. In this case they could be presented as a clustered bar chart (Figure 3.5). When presenting data in this way (as percentages), you should include the *denominator* for each group (total sample size), as giving percentages alone can be misleading if the groups contained very different numbers of subjects.

It is possible to use different colours to distinguish between the different groups, but as with pie charts, it is best to use different shades of the same colour to represent different groups. This has been done in Figure 3.5.

Note that the bars and vertical scale now represent the percentage of cases rather than the actual number (i.e. the relative frequency). The relative frequency scale has been used rather than the count scale as this enables comparisons to be made between the groups when the numbers in each group differ, as in this example with parity. If the relative frequency scale is used, it is recommended good practice to report the total sample size for each group in the legend. In this way, given the total sample size and relative frequency (from the height of the bars) it is possible to work out the actual numbers of mothers with the different types of delivery. An alternative method would

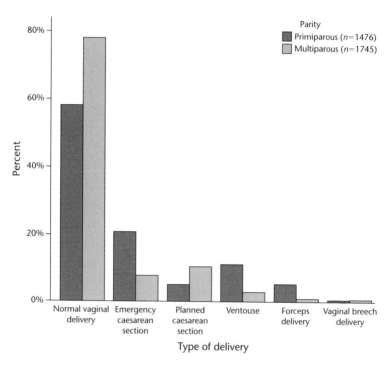

Figure 3.5 Self-reported type of delivery by parity for mothers at 8 weeks postnatally.[1]

be to display the data for primiparous and multiparous women separately as in Figure 3.6. However, this would be a poor method of display since the purpose in plotting the data together is to compare the primiparous and multiparous women. This comparison is much less easy with Figure 3.6 and so the data should be plotted together as in Figure 3.5.

The clustered bar chart in Figure 3.5 clearly shows that there is a difference in the self-reported type of delivery experienced by first time mothers compared to mothers who already have a child. Primiparous mothers are less likely to report a normal vaginal delivery and more likely to report having an emergency caesarean section than multiparous women. If the actual counts had been used on the vertical axis, then this difference in the proportions between the two groups would not have been as obvious because of the different sizes of the two groups (e.g. 1476 primiparous vs. 1745 multiparous women).

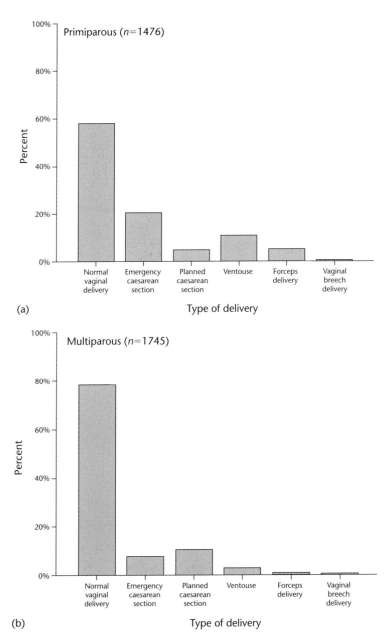

Figure 3.6 Self-reported type of delivery by parity for mothers at 8 weeks postnatally ($n = 3221$) – this method of display is not recommended:[1](a) primiparous and (b) multiparous.

3.6 Stacked bar charts

As the number of groups to be compared increases, a clustered bar chart can quickly become very busy and obscure patterns within the data. When the number of groups to be compared becomes greater than three or four, a better type of bar chart is the stacked bar chart, where the groups are arranged on the horizontal axis and the variable being compared between the groups is arranged on the vertical axis.

As part of the postal questionnaire survey of new mothers, the women were asked their age and what method of feeding they were using. As before, these data can be classified in two ways, by maternal age and method of infant feeding enabling the feeding method chosen to be compared between mothers of different ages as in Table 3.4. These data may be plotted using a stacked bar chart (Figure 3.7). As the comparison of interest is between women of different ages, age should be on the horizontal axis and method of feeding on the vertical axis. From Figure 3.7 it can easily be seen that there is a tendency for increasing breast-feeding as maternal age increases, with the exception of the oldest mothers. Note that the vertical axis has been scaled, from 0 to 100, to represent the percentage in each age group who use a particular feeding method.

Table 3.4 Feeding method by maternal age for all women ($n = 3211$)[1]

Maternal age (years)	n	Breast milk only (%)	Breast and formula milk (%)	Formula milk only (%)
<20	270	5.6	6.7	87.8
20–24	574	11.3	7.1	81.5
25–29	1006	17.9	9.4	72.7
30–34	915	25.1	14.3	60.5
35–39	350	27.4	18.0	54.6
40+	96	24.0	12.5	63.5
Totals	3211	19.0	11.2	69.8

As with clustered bar charts it is good practice to include the numbers in each category being compared. In addition the different feeding categories have been shaded, rather than using either colour or pattern.

The nice feature of stacked bar charts, which is lost in clustered bar charts, is that it reminds the reader that since percentages are constrained to sum to 100, if one category increases, others perforce must decrease. However, as discussed in Chapter 2, one disadvantage of stacked bar charts

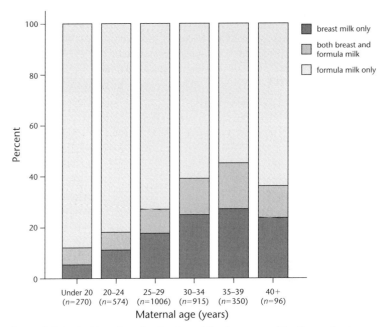

Figure 3.7 Stacked bar chart showing the relative frequency of feeding methods between the different age groups.[1]

is that it is difficult to compare intermediate categories such as the mixed feeding category (both breast & formula milk) in Figure 3.7. In general clustered bar charts are preferable.

Summary of the main points when displaying categorical data

- Categorical data can be displayed using either pie charts or bar charts.
- Bar charts are preferable to pie charts.
- Use pie charts only for displaying one set of proportions.
- Use clustered bar charts to display two or more sets of proportions.
- Always include the total number of subjects; for cluster or stacked bar charts always include the number in each group.
- Never use three-dimensional bar charts or pie charts, they are difficult to read and can be misleading.
- Different shades of the same colour are best for distinguishing between different categories. Colours and patterns to distinguish between different groups should be used with caution.
- Discrete or count data can be displayed using bar charts.

References

1 O'Cathain A, Walters S, Nicholl JP, Thomas KJ, Kirkham M. Use of evidence based
   leaflets to promote infomred choice in maternity care: randomised controlled trial
   in everyday practice. *British Medical Journal* 2002;**324**:643–6.
2 Ehrenberg ASC. *A primer in data reduction.* Chichester: John Wiley & Sons; 2000.

Chapter 4 **Displaying quantitative data**

This chapter will describe the basic graphs available for displaying quantitative data. As described in Chapter 1 quantitative data can be either counted or continuous. *Count* data are also known as discrete data and as the name implies occur when the data can be counted, such as the number of children in a family or the number of visits to a GP in a year. *Continuous* data are data that can be measured and in principle they can take any value on the scale on which they are measured; they are limited only by the precision of the scale of measurement and examples include height, weight and blood pressure.

4.1 Count data

Count data can only take whole numbers and the best method to display them is using a bar chart. As with categorical data, an initial step is to add up the number of observations in each category and express them as percentages of the total sample size. For example, Table 4.1 shows data from an investigation by Campbell of the effect of environmental temperature on the number of deaths attributed to Sudden Infant Death Syndrome (SIDS).[1] The table summarises the numbers of deaths, in England and Wales, from SIDS each day over a 5-year period (1979–1983) ($n = 1819$ days). Figure 4.1 displays these data using a bar chart. On the horizontal axis are the number of deaths per day, going from a minimum of 0 deaths per day to a maximum of 16 deaths per day, while on the vertical axis is the frequency with which these occur during this 5-year period. The vertical scale for this graph is the frequency; this could easily be rescaled to percentages. As discussed in Chapter 3 there are advantages to both types of scale and the shape of the resultant chart will not be affected by the choice of scale. Use of the percentage scale facilitates the comparison of groups. For example, if it was of interest to compare England and Wales with Scotland, the smaller number for Scotland would make comparison more difficult if the frequency scale were used.

Table 4.1 Number of deaths from SIDS per day,
England and Wales, 1979–1983

Number of deaths per day	Number of days (%)
0	121 (6.7)
1	277 (15.2)
2	330 (18.1)
3	307 (16.9)
4	270 (14.8)
5	205 (11.3)
6	127 (7.0)
7	89 (4.9)
8	45 (2.5)
9	20 (1.1)
10	14 (0.8)
11	8 (0.4)
12	4 (0.2)
13	1 (0.1)
14	–
15	–
16	9 (0.1)
Total	1819 (100.0)

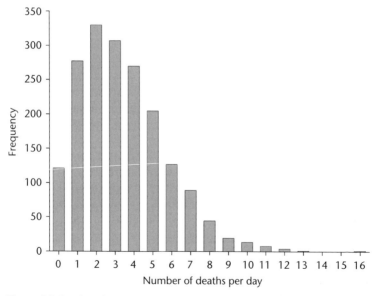

Figure 4.1 Bar chart showing the distribution of number of sudden infant deaths per day for England and Wales, 1979–1983 (n = 1819).[1]

Count data are ordered in that there is a natural ordering to the groups: 2 children in a family is more than 1, and 3 is more than 2 and so on. Thus, a bar chart displays the shape of the distribution of the data. This would not be obtained from a pie chart. Pie charts should not be used for count data as they make no use of the additional information that arises from the ordering of the data.

4.2 Graphs for continuous data

A variety of graphs exists for plotting continuous data. The simplest graphs are *dotplots* and *stem and leaf* plots and they both display all the data. In addition there are other graphs which provide useful summaries of the data such as *histograms* and *box-and-whisker* plots.

4.3 Dotplots

A basic principle for displaying data is 'above all else display the data'.[2] Dotplots are perfect for following this maxim as each point represents a value for a single individual. They are one of the simplest ways of displaying all the data. As part of a study examining the cost effectiveness of specialist leg ulcer clinics compared to standard district nursing care participants were asked their height.[3] Figure 4.2a shows dot plots of the heights of the participants. Each dot represents the value for an individual and is plotted along a vertical axis, which in this case, represents height in metres. Data for several groups can be plotted alongside each other for comparison; Figure 4.2b shows these data plotted by sex and in this case the differences in height between men and women can be clearly seen.

4.4 Stem and leaf plots

Another simple way of showing all the data is the stem and leaf plot. Each data point is divided into two parts, a stem and a leaf; the leaf is usually the last digit and the stem is the other part of the number. For example, for a height of 1.58 m, the leaf would be 8 and the stem would be 1.5. Each data point in the sample is thus divided and the results displayed in the form of a stem and leaf plot. There is a separate line for each different stem value, but within particular stem values the individual leaf values are arranged on the same line. The stem is on the left of the plot and the leaves are on the right. In addition the number of data points in each stem can also be displayed on the left. It is easiest to understand by means of an example.

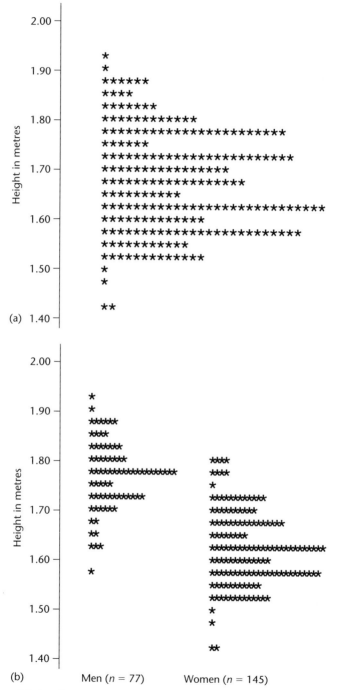

Figure 4.2 Dot plots of height of patients in the leg ulcer trial in metres ($n = 222$):[3] (a) for all patients and (b) by sex.

The heights, in metres, of the first 10 men enrolled into the leg ulcer study are as follows:

1.88, 1.78, 1.73, 1.93, 1.85, 1.75, 1.78, 1.78, 1.70, 1.65

Taking the first number of the series above, the stem is 1.8, the leaf is 8 and the frequency for that row is 1:

Frequency	Stem	Leaf
1	**1.8**	**8**

Taking the next height, 1.78:

Frequency	Stem	Leaf
1	**1.7**	**8**
1	1.8	8

And the next height, 1.73:

Frequency	Stem	Leaf
2	**1.7**	**83**
1	1.8	8

And so on....

Frequency	Stem	Leaf
1	1.6	5
6	1.7	835880
2	1.8	85
1	1.9	3

Figure 4.3 shows a stem and leaf plot for the heights of all 77 men.

However, in this plot it can be seen that there is a lot of bunching particularly for the 1.7 stem. In this case and for other plots where there are few stems and many individuals in each stem, the stems can be further divided, such that each stem line represents a smaller interval. For the present case, the stems can be divided to represent intervals of 5 cm as in Figure 4.4.

In all the stem and leaf plots above, the leaves are arranged in the order of how the values occur in the data series and these are known as 'as they come' stem and leaf plots. However, we recommend ordering the values in

Frequency	Stem	Leaf
1	1.5	7
7	1.6	5833385
42	1.7	835880388388838880335533800088838588833350
25	1.8	85353333588880350000003800
2	1.9	31

Figure 4.3 Stem and leaf plot of the height of the male leg ulcer patients, with stems of size 10 cm, $n = 77$.[3]

Frequency	Stem	Leaf
1	1.55-	7
3	1.60-	333
4	1.65-	5885
18	1.70-	303330333300033303
24	1.75-	858888888888558888858885
15	1.80-	333330300000300
10	1.85-	8555888858
1	1.90-	31

Figure 4.4 Stem and leaf plot of the height of the male leg ulcer patients, with stems of size 5 cm, $n = 77$.[3]

Frequency	Stem	Leaf
1	1.55-	7
3	1.60-	333
4	1.65-	5588
18	1.70-	000000333333333333
24	1.75-	555558888888888888888888
15	1.80-	000000003333333
10	1.85-	5555888888
1	1.90-	13

Figure 4.5 Ordered stem and leaf plot of the height of the male leg ulcer patients, $n = 77$.[3]

the individual stems as shown in Figure 4.5. The ordered stem and leaf plot contains more information. For example given the sample size of the data set it is a simple matter to work out the median. The median value is the middle value when the data are ordered, such that half of the observations lie below this value and half lie above it and is one of the basic measures of location.[4] In this case there are 77 observations and thus the median is the 39th value (when the data are ordered), as 38 observations lie below this point and 38 lie above. Looking at Figure 4.5 it can be seen that the 39th value occurs in stem 1.75 and the leaf value corresponding to the 39th value is 8. Thus the median for these data is a height of 1.78 m.

A further point to note about these data is the digit preference exhibited; all the leaves are either, 0, 1, 3, 5 or 8. The reason is that height was not measured in the study but provided by the patients. As most were elderly they gave height information in feet and inches which was then converted to metric. This sort of detailed examination of the data would not be possible from a histogram (see next section). A stem and leaf plot resembles a histogram turned over onto its side. The advantage of a stem and leaf plot over a histogram is that not only does it show the frequency in each stem but that it retains the individual values of the data.

4.5 Histograms

A common method for displaying continuous data is a *histogram*. In order to construct a histogram the data range is divided into several non-overlapping equally sized bins (categories) and the number of observations falling into each bin counted. The categories are then displayed on the horizontal axis (*X*-axis) and the frequencies displayed on the vertical axis (*Y*-axis), as in Figure 4.6. As with pie charts and bar charts the area of each bin is proportional to the number of observations in the bin. Occasionally the percentages in each category are displayed on the *Y*-axis rather than the frequencies and it is important that if this is done, the total number of observations that the percentages are based upon must be included in the graph. The choice of number of categories is important as using too few categories results in much important information being lost (Figure 4.6a); too many and any patterns are obscured by too much detail (Figure 4.6b). Although there are no hard and fast rules about the appropriate number of bins, usually between 5 and 15 categories will be enough to gain an idea of the distribution of the data (Figure 4.6c).

From Figure 4.6c the different peaks for men and women can be clearly seen. With these data it is better to display the heights for men and women in separate histograms as in Figure 4.7. However, when using histograms to display data from several groups, it is important to ensure that both the axes are on the same scale for all charts. In doing this, it is then possible to compare directly between groups. If there are different number of subjects in each of the groups then it is important that percentages or relative frequencies are displayed on the vertical (*Y*-axis) and not the frequencies. For the height data displayed below, several points are immediately

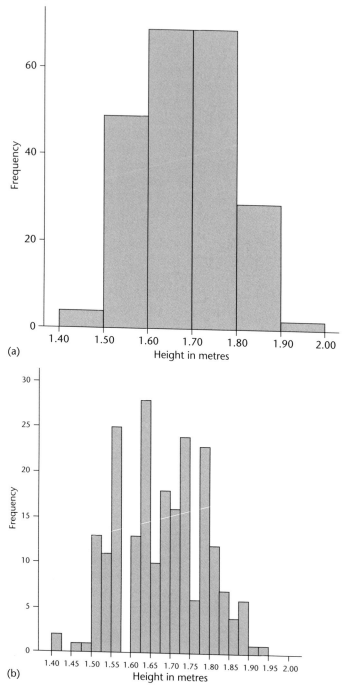

Figure 4.6 Histograms of height for leg ulcer patients:[3] ($n = 222$) (a) with only 6 categories, (b) with 22 categories and (c) with 9 categories (see over).

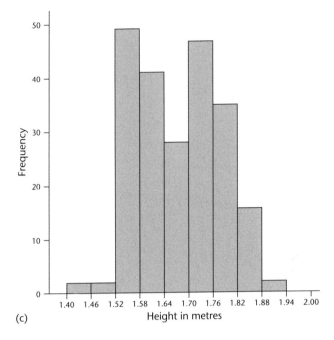

(c)

Figure 4.6 (*Continued.*)

obvious: there are more women than men; and the peak for men occurs at a greater height than for women (about 1.80 m compared to 1.62 m).

The bins or intervals on the horizontal X-axis of the histogram can be labelled in a variety of ways. The bars may be labelled by using the mid-point of the corresponding interval, or by having a label at the start (or end) of the interval as in Figure 4.6. For histograms, we recommend that you label the horizontal axis, at the start (or end) of each interval, since with this method it is easier to work out the width of the interval (as in Figure 4.6). Some intermediate interval labels can be omitted, to avoid cluttering up the scale, without any noticeably loss of clarity as in Figure 4.6b.

A useful feature of a histogram is that it is possible to assess the distributional form of the data; in particular whether the data are approximately Normally distributed, or are skewed. The *Normal distribution* (sometimes known as the Gaussian distribution) is one of the fundamental distributions of statistics, and the histogram of Normally distributed data will have a classic 'bell' shape, with a peak in the middle and symmetrical tails, such as that for height for women in Figure 4.7b. *Skewed* data are data which are not symmetrical; positively skewed data have a peak at lower values and a

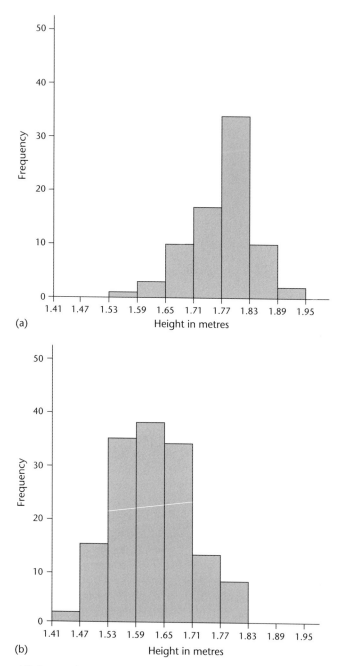

Figure 4.7 Separate histograms for the heights of men and women:[3] (a) for men ($n = 77$) and (b) for women ($n = 145$).

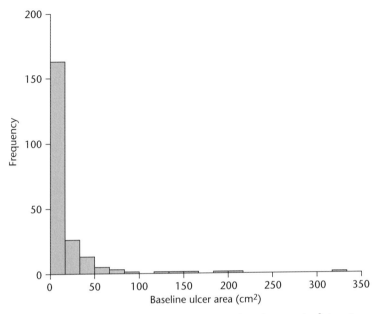

Figure 4.8 Positively skewed data – histogram of baseline ulcer area (cm^2) from leg ulcer trial (n = 217).[3]

long tail of higher values (Figure 4.8) while conversely negatively skewed data have a long left-hand tail at lower values, with a peak at higher values (see Figure 4.9).

Histograms are similar to bar charts in that the variable of interest is displayed on the horizontal axis (X-axis) and the frequencies are displayed on the vertical axis (Y-axis). However bar charts are used for discontinuous data, where the categories are entirely separate while histograms are used for continuous data. Thus bar charts have gaps between the categories on the horizontal axis in order to emphasise that the categories are completely separate, whereas there are no spaces in between the bins for a histogram, as the width of these bins can be set by the investigator.

The count data, for the number of deaths from SIDS per day, in Table 4.1 could also be displayed as a histogram. This is because there are a large number of categories (14) of deaths per day and it is reasonable to treat such discrete count data as if they were continuous, at least as far as the statistical analysis goes. However we would recommend count data should be displayed using bar charts as opposed to histograms, as the gaps between the bars will emphasise that the categories represent discrete whole numbers and cannot take intermediate values (e.g. it is not possible to have 1.3 SIDS per day).

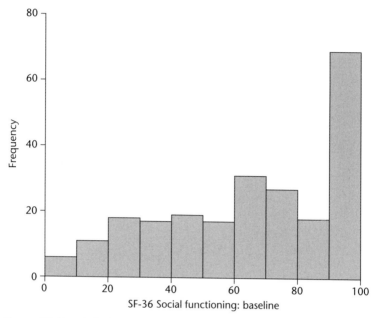

Figure 4.9 Negatively skewed data – histogram of baseline social functioning from leg ulcer trial (*n* = 233).[3]

4.6 Box–whisker plots

Another extremely useful method of plotting continuous data is *a box-and-whisker* or *box plot*. This is described in detail in Figure 4.10. As with dot plots, box plots can be particularly useful for comparing the distribution of the data across several groups.

The box contains the middle 50% of the data, with lowest 25% of the data lying below it and the highest 25% of the data lying above it. In fact the upper and lower edges represent a particular quantity called the inter-quartile range. The horizontal line in the middle of the box represents the median value as described in Section 4.4. The whiskers extend to the largest and smallest values excluding the outlying values. The outlying values are defined as those values more than 1.5 box lengths from the upper or lower edges, and are represented as the dots outside the whiskers. Figure 4.10 shows box plots of the heights of the men and women in the leg ulcer trial.

Similar to dot plots, the gender differences in height are immediately obvious from this plot and this illustrates the main advantage of the box plot over histograms when looking at multiple groups. Differences in the

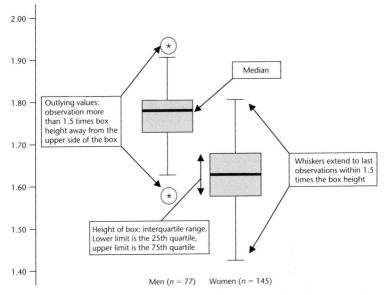

Figure 4.10 Annotated box plots of height for the leg ulcer patients by sex, showing what each of the items displayed mean.[3]

distributions of data between groups are much easier to spot with box plots than with histograms. As a result of what they display (median, inter-quartile range, spread) they provide a good summary of the data and are more useful than dot plots for larger datasets, where a dot plot would look rather busy.

Summary

- Display univariate count data using bar charts as opposed to histograms unless the number of categories is large enough to be treated as approximately continuous, in which case a histogram can be used.
- Always display continuous data as dotplots if the sample size per group is low (≤100 subjects).
- For univariate data a stem and leaf plot can be useful since all the data are available in the chart.
- Use histograms to show the distribution of single variables.
- To compare groups, for larger samples (say >50 subjects per group) use box–whisker plots.

References

1 Campbell MJ. Time series regression for counts: an investigation into the relationship between Sudden Infant Death Syndrome and environmental temperature. *Journal of the Royal Statistical Society, Series A* 1994;**157**:191–208.

2 Tufte ER. *The visual display of quantitative information.* Cheshire, Connecticut: Graphics Press; 1983.

3 Morrell CJ, Walters SJ, Dixon S, Collins K, Brereton LML, Peters J, et al. Cost effectiveness of community leg ulcer clinic: randomised controlled trial. *British Medical Journal* 1998;**316**:1487–91.

4 Freeman JV, Julious S. Describing and summarising data. SCOPE 2005. Vol 14(3).

Chapter 5 **Displaying the relationship between two continuous variables**

5.1 Introduction

This chapter will concentrate on methods for displaying the relation-ship between two continuous variables. A large proportion of statisti-cal analyses are conducted to investigate the relationship between two variables for a particular group of subjects. Such analyses have several purposes:

– To assess whether the two variables are associated (correlation).
– To enable the value of one variable to be predicted from any known value of the other variable (regression). One variable is regarded as a response to the other explanatory variable.
– To assess the amount of agreement between the values of the two variables. Most commonly this situation arises in the comparison of alternative ways of measuring or assessing the same thing.
– To diagnose of a disease or a condition (present/absent) using the results of a test with a continuous measurement scale.

The statistical method for assessing the linear association between two continuous variables is known as *correlation*. The method for predicting the value of one continuous variable from another is known as *regression*. As correlation and regression are often presented together it is easy to get the impression that they are inseparable. In fact, they have distinct purposes and it is relatively rare that one is genuinely interested in performing both analyses on the same set of data.

However, when preparing to conduct either analysis it is essential to construct a scatter diagram of the values of one of the variables against the values of the other variable. By drawing a scatter diagram one can see immediately whether or not there is any visual evidence of a straight line or linear association between the two variables.

5.2 Correlation

Figure 5.1 shows a scatter diagram of the systolic and diastolic blood pressure amongst 96 adults with carotid artery disease aged 42–89 years prior to

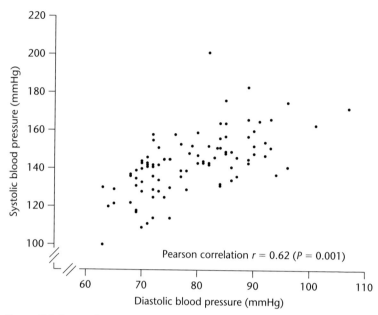

Figure 5.1 Scatter diagram of systolic vs. diastolic blood pressure for 96 patients with carotid artery disease.[1]

surgery. The data come from a randomised-controlled trial which aimed to compare outcomes after two forms of surgery (carotid angioplasty (PTA) and endarterectomy (CEA)) in patients with symptomatic carotid artery disease.[1] There appears to be some association between the values of the two variables; we can see that there is a tendency for patients with higher diastolic blood pressure to have higher systolic blood pressure.

With correlation, it is not important which variable is plotted on the X (horizontal) axis and which is plotted in the Y (vertical) axis as what is of interest is to see whether as the values of one variable change, the values of the other variable change as well. In this example the systolic and diastolic blood pressure variables could be plotted on either the X or Y-axis. Either variable could cause or influence the other. In contrast, if we were interested in the relationship between height and weight, then as height to some extent determines weight and not the other way round (the weight a person is does not determine their height) it is recommended to plot height on the X-axis and weight on the Y-axis.

The degree of association, between systolic and diastolic blood pressures in this example, can be measured using *the correlation coefficient*. The standard method called *Pearson's correlation coefficient* leads to a quantity called *r* which can take any value from −1 to +1. This measures the degree of straight line association between the values of the two variables. It is positive if higher values of one variable are associated with higher values of the other and negative if one variable tends to be low as the other gets higher. A correlation of around zero indicates that there is no linear relation between the values of the two variables. Clearly, the systolic and diastolic blood pressure variables in Figure 5.1 are positively correlated, and the correlation coefficient is *r* = 0.62. Technical details on how to calculate correlation coefficients are given in Chapter 9 of Campbell, Machin and Walters.[2]

Figure 5.2 shows the same data, but with the origin (systolic blood pressure of 0 mmHg and diastolic blood pressure of 0 mmHg), included for both the *X* and *Y*-axis. In this graph there is a large amount of blank space, since no patient in this sample has a diastolic blood pressure below 60 mmHg or a systolic blood pressure below 100 mmHg. This graph clearly shows that the relationship between systolic and diastolic blood pressure is only valid, in this sample, for a limited range of diastolic blood pressures between 60 and 110 mmHg. Rather than waste space, the scales on either the horizontal

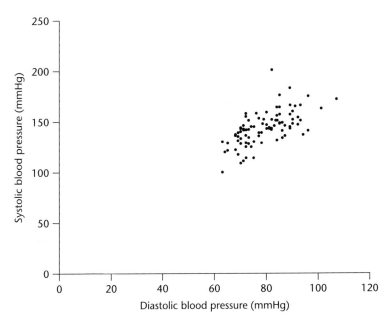

Figure 5.2 Scatter diagram of systolic vs. diastolic blood pressure for 96 patients with carotid artery disease with zero origin for both axes.[1]

or vertical axes or both axes can be truncated to reflect the actual range of observations for the two variables in the sample. In these circumstances, as Figure 5.1 illustrates, it is good practice to notch or score the truncated axis with two parallel line symbols '//' to indicate that the origin or zero value for the axis has been omitted.

If the sample consisted of different subgroups for whom it was thought that the correlation might differ then it is possible to use different symbols and colours for the different subgroups in the scatter diagram. However, if colour is used, care should be taken as different colours can appear the same when photocopied. For example, the blood pressure data in Figure 5.1 relates to 64 men and 32 women. By using different symbols or different colours to distinguish between men and women it is possible to see visually whether the relationship between the two blood pressure variables is the same in the two groups (Figure 5.3). From Figure 5.3, this appears to be the case.

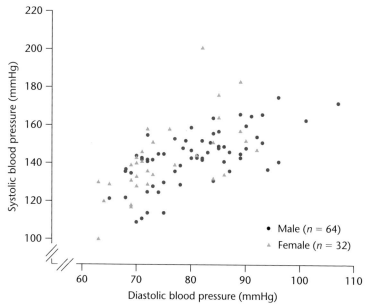

Figure 5.3 Scatter diagram of systolic vs. diastolic blood pressure for 96 patients with carotid artery disease by sex.[1]

Correlation is often used as an exploratory method for investigating the interrelationships among several continuous variables. Simpson describes a prospective study in which 98 pre-term infants were given a series of tests shortly after they were born, in an attempt to predict their outcome after

1 year.[3] Measurements recorded include maternal age (in years), birthweight (kilograms) and the gestational age (weeks) of the baby.

The correlations between all possible pairs of variables can be done by means of a correlation matrix as in Table 5.1. In this, the correlation coefficients are shown in a triangular display similar to the charts in road atlases showing the distances between pairs of towns. The graphical equivalent, in Figure 5.4 is

Table 5.1 Correlation matrix for gestation, maternal age and birthweight for 98 pre-term babies[3]

	Gestation (weeks)	Maternal age (years)	Birthweight (kg)
Gestation (weeks)	1.00		
Maternal age (years)	0.01	1.00	
Birthweight (kg)	0.81	0.02	1.00

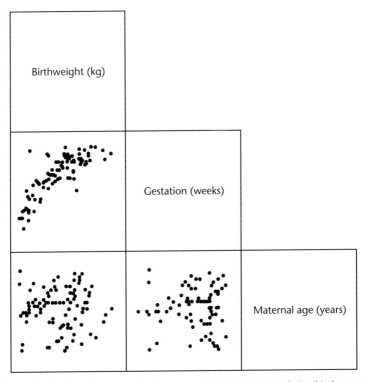

Figure 5.4 Scatter diagram matrix showing each of the two-way relationship between maternal age, birthweight and gestation in 98 premature babies.[3]

even better. Here it is clear that there is a strong correlation between birth-weight and gestation age, and no relation between either birthweight and maternal age, or gestational age and maternal age.

5.3 Regression

When it is plausible that the values of one variable exert an influence on the values of the other variable a technique known as regression can be used. In this chapter we shall only consider the simple case of a single continuous explanatory (independent) variable and a single continuous outcome (dependent) variable. Further methods of displaying the results of a regression analysis with more than one explanatory variable are given in Chapter 7. Often it is of interest to quantify the relationship between the two variables, and given a particular value of the explanatory variable for an individual, to predict the value of the outcome variable. As with correlation, these data should be plotted using a scatter diagram. However, unlike correlation it is essential that the explanatory variable (the one exerting the influence) is plotted on the X-axis and the outcome variable (the one being influenced) is plotted on the Y-axis.

Figure 5.5 shows the birthweight and gestational age of 98 pre-term babies in the Simpson study. As birthweight, to some extent, is influenced by gestational age it is important to plot gestational age on the X-axis and birthweight on the Y-axis. Using regression, birthweight can be predicted from gestational age. The response variable is always plotted on the vertical, or Y, axis and the predictor variable on the horizontal, or X, axis as illustrated in Figure 5.5.

When displaying the scatter diagram for a regression analysis the regression line should be plotted. The regression equation can also be included. The regression equation is given by the formula $y = a + bx$. Briefly the intercept, a, is the point at which the line crosses the Y-axis (i.e. when the value of the x variable is zero) and the slope, b, gives the average change in the y variable for a single unit change in the x variable. The slope coefficient for gestational age is 0.135 kg and this suggests that for every unit or one week increase in gestation, then birthweight increases by 0.135 kg. The intercept coefficient is -2.66. In most medical applications the value of the intercept will have no practical meaning, as the x variable cannot be anywhere near zero. The value of r^2 or R^2 is often quoted in published articles and indicates the proportion (sometimes expressed as a percentage) of the total variability of the outcome variable that is explained by the regression model fitted. In this case 66% of the total variability in birthweight is explained by gestation.

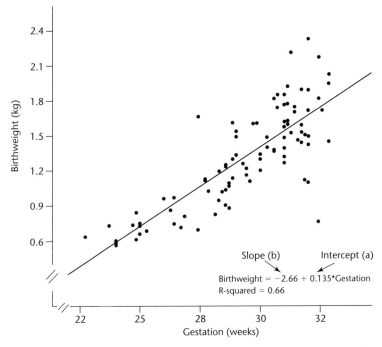

Figure 5.5 Relationship between gestation and birthweight in 98 pre-term babies.[3]

Note that the regression model should not be used to predict outside of the range of observations. In addition, it should not be assumed that just because an equation has been produced it means that x causes y. In the present example, there may also be other factors that exert an influence upon birthweight, such as maternal smoking and maternal diabetes (see Chapter 9 of Campbell, Machin and Walters for more details).[2]

5.4 Lowess smoothing plots

Looking at the scatter diagram in Figure 5.5, there is a suggestion that the relationship between birthweight and gestational age may be non-linear, particularly for gestations above 30 weeks. The dots suggest that a quadratic relationship may not be unreasonable for these data. Graphically, this relationship can be investigated using a local weighted regression analysis.[4] Plotting a smooth curve through a set of data points using this statistical technique is called a *Lowess Curve*. Lowess curves are a useful way of visually exploring the relationship between two continuous variables as the shape of the curve at any point along the axes is determined by the data nearest to it and not by all the data, thus they can be sensitive to small localised changes in the way that a simple linear regression line is not. Thus they can hint at subtle changes that would not be obvious from a linear regression.

Exact details of how the curve is fitted may be found in Cleveland, but briefly, Lowess curves work by fitting a low degree polynomial model to localised subsets of the data to build up a function that describes the deterministic part (i.e. contains no random elements) of the variation in the data, point by point. In order to fit a Lowess curve it is necessary to specify the amount of data used in each localised subset (bandwidth) and the weight to be given to each point fitted in the model. Many of the details of this method, such as the degree of the polynomial model and the weights, are flexible. So, unlike linear regression there is no unique Lowess curve for a given set of data. Figure 5.6 shows the scatter diagram of the data with the Lowess curve fitted using a 'bandwidth' of 50% of the data points and uniform weight for each of the data points for the curve.

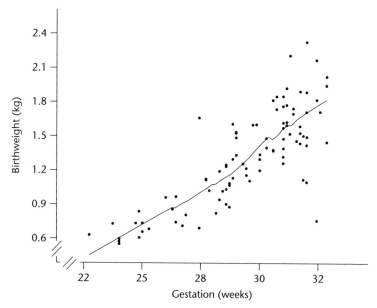

Figure 5.6 Relationship between gestation and birthweight, with locally weighted regression line or Lowess curve, in 98 pre-term babies with a bandwidth of 50% of the data and uniform weights.[3]

The Lowess curve in Figure 5.6 suggests a kink or slight curvature to the prediction of birthweight between 30 and 32 weeks gestation but overall the curve does not provide any strong evidence of a non-linear relationship between birthweight and gestation in this sample. So we can therefore assume a linear relationship between birthweight and gestation and the model presented in Figure 5.5 is not unreasonable for these data. The usefulness of Lowess curves is further explored in Chapter 8.

5.5 Assessing agreement between two continuous variables

The most common situation when assessing the amount of agreement between the values of two variables arises in the comparison of alternative ways of measuring or assessing the same thing. Most measurements (e.g. blood pressure, height or weight) are not precise and are subject to measurement error or variability over time or both. As a result of these uncertainties, there are usually a variety of measurement techniques available and studies to compare the level of agreement between two methods of measurement are common. The aim of these studies is usually to see if the methods agree well enough for one method to replace the other, or perhaps for the two methods to be used interchangeably. The same considerations apply to studies comparing two observers using a single measurement method. We need to define what we mean by agreement between the two methods, and the degree of agreement. The best approach to this type of problem and data is to analyse the differences between the measurements by the two methods (or two observers) on each subject.

The graphical methods available for displaying data from method comparison studies will be illustrated with data comparing two observers using the same assessment checklist. Two clinicians (Reviewer 1 and Reviewer 2) were asked to rate the overall quality of care, using a standardised assessment checklist, as described in the hospital notes of 48 patients with chronic obstructive pulmonary disease (COPD) at a particular hospital.[5] Quality of care was rated on a 10-point scale with a score of 1 indicating poor care and a score of 10 indicating excellent care. Figure 5.7 shows a scatter diagram of the data. If the observers agreed exactly then all the points would lie on the line of equality (a line with a 45 degree slope passing through the origins of the X and Y-axis). However, it can be seen that although some of the data are near to the line of equality, there are several patients where the two scores differ considerably.

For several of the patients' notes, the two reviewers rated the quality of care with the same combination of scores, for example there were six patients where Reviewer 1 rated the care as 9 and Reviewer 2 rated the care as an 8.

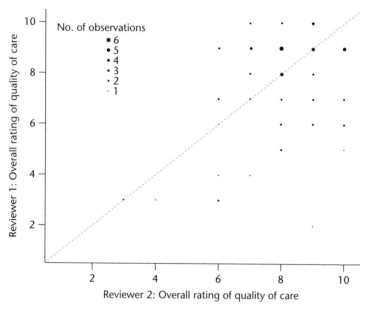

Figure 5.7 Scatter diagram of two observers (Reviewer 1 vs. Reviewer 2) ratings of the overall quality of care score from the medical notes score of 48 patients with COPD with line of equality.[5]

These overlapping data pairs would be shown as only one point or combination on the scatter graph. This is slightly misleading as there are actually six data pairs with this combination of reviewer scores. This problem can be solved by having different sized markers for the various pairs of scores, with the size of the marker relative to the number of data values with this combination of reviewer scores.

5.6 Bland–Altman plots

An alternative, more informative plot has been proposed by Bland and Altman as shown in Figure 5.9.[6] Here the difference in scores between the two reviewers (Reviewer 1–Reviewer 2) is plotted against their average. Three things are readily observable with this type of plot:

1 The size of the differences between reviewers.
2 The distribution of these differences about zero.
3 Whether the differences are related to the size of the measurement (for this purpose the average of the two reviewers' scores acts as the best estimate of the true unknown value).

How well do the two methods (or observers in our example) agree? We could simply quote the mean difference and standard deviation of the differences (SD_{diff}). However, it is more useful to use these to construct a range of values which would be expected to cover the agreement between the methods for most subjects[7] and the *95% limits of agreement* are defined as the mean difference $\pm 2SD_{diff}$. For the current example the mean difference is -0.44 (SD 2.06) and the limits of agreement are given by -4.56 to 3.68. These are shown in Figure 5.8 as dotted lines, along with the mean difference of -0.44. As with plot 5.7 the size of the dots on the plot are proportional to the number of observations that have contributed to the dots.

In Figure 5.8, only 2 out of 48 (4%) of the observations are outside the 95% limits of agreement. However, there is considerable variability in the difference in quality of care scores between the two reviewers, even though the mean difference is small (-0.44). The limits of agreement are wide, almost 5 points in either direction, which is half the quality of care scale

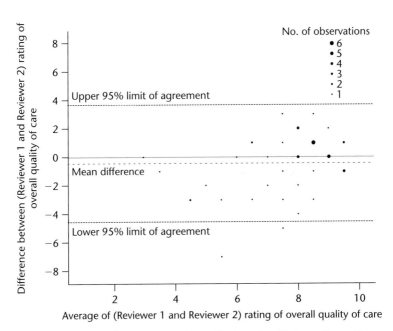

Figure 5.8 Difference between two reviewers (Reviewer 1 vs. Reviewer 2) overall quality of care score plotted average quality care score based on the rating of the medical notes of 48 patients with COPD, plus the observed mean difference and 95% limits of agreement.[5]

range. This suggests that there is poor agreement between two observers using the same standardised checklist to assess overall quality of care.

5.7 ROC curves for diagnostic tests

Another common situation when we want to display two continuous variables is when developing a screening or diagnostic test for the diagnosis of a disease or a condition using the results of a test which uses either an ordinal or continuous measurement scale. For every diagnostic procedure it is important to know its sensitivity (the probability that a person with the disease will test positive) and its specificity (the probability that a person without the disease will test negative). These questions can be answered only if it is known what the 'true' diagnosis is. This may be determined by biopsy or an expensive and risky procedure such as angiography for heart disease. In other situations it may be by 'expert' opinion. Such tests provide the so-called 'gold standard'.

When a diagnostic test produces a continuous measurement, then a convenient diagnostic cut-off must be selected to calculate the sensitivity and specificity of the test. For example, a positive diagnostic result of 'hypertension' is a diastolic blood pressure greater than 90 mmHg; whereas for 'anaemia', a haemoglobin level less than 12 g/dl is used as the cut-off.

Johnson et al. looked at 106 patients about to undergo an operation for acute pancreatitis.[8] Before the operation, they were assessed for risk using a score known as the APACHE (Acute Physiology and Chronic Health Evaluation) II score. APACHE II was designed to measure the severity of disease for patients (aged 16 years or more) admitted to intensive care units. It ranges in value from 0 to 27. The authors also wanted to compare this score with a newly devised one, the APACHE_O which included a measure of obesity. The convention is that if the APACHE II is at least 8 the patient is at high risk of severe complications. Table 5.2 shows the results using this cut-off value.

Table 5.2 Number of subjects above and below 8 of the APACHE II score severity of complication[8]

APACHE II	Complication after operation		
	Mild	Severe	Total
<8	8	5	13
≥8	5	22	27
Total	13	27	40

For the data in Table 5.2 the sensitivity is 22/27 = 0.81, or 81%, and the specificity is 8/13 = 0.62, or 62%.

In the above example, we need not have chosen APACHE II = 8 as the cut-off value. For each possible value (from 0 to 27) there is a corresponding sensitivity and specificity. We can display these calculations by graphing the sensitivity on the Y-axis (vertical) and the false positive rate (1 − specificity) on the X-axis (horizontal) for all possible cut-off values of the diagnostic test (from 0 to 27, for the current example). The resulting curve is known as the *relative (or receiver) operating characteristic curve* (ROC). The ROC for the data of Johnson et al. (2004) are shown in Figure 5.9 for the APACHE II and APACHE_O data.

A perfect diagnostic test would be one with no false negative (i.e. sensitivity of 1) or false positive (specificity of 1) results and would be represented by a line that started at the origin and went vertically straight up the Y-axis to a sensitivity of 1, and then horizontally across to a false positive rate of 1. A test that produces false positive results at the same rate as true positive results would produce an ROC on the diagonal line $y = x$. Any reasonable diagnostic test will display an ROC curve in the upper left triangle of Figure 5.9.

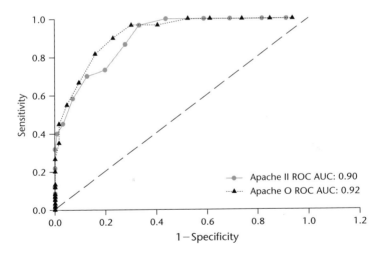

Figure 5.9 Receiver–operator curve for Apache_O and Apache II data from 106 patients with acute pancreatitis.[8]

The selection of an optimal combination of sensitivity and specificity for a particular test requires an analysis of the relative medical consequences and costs of false positive and false negative classifications. An angiogram is rarely used for screening patients for suspected heart disease as it is a difficult and expensive procedure, and carries a non-negligible risk to the patient. An alternative test such as an exercise test is usually tried and only if it is positive would angiography then be carried out. If the exercise test is negative then the next stage would be to carry out biochemical tests, and if these turned out positive, once again angiography could be performed.

5.8 Analysis of ROC curves

As already indicated, a perfect diagnostic test would be represented by a line that started at the origin, travelled up the Y-axis to a sensitivity of 1, then across the ceiling to an X-axis (false positive) value of 1. The area under this ROC curve, termed the AUC, is then the total area of the panel; that is, $1 \times 1 = 1$. The AUC can be used as a measure of the performance of a diagnostic test against the ideal and may also be used to compare different tests. When more than one laboratory test is available for the same clinical problem one can compare ROC curves, by plotting both on the same figure as in Figure 5.9 and comparing the area under the curve. In the example of Figure 5.9, the two tests are not 'perfect' but it is readily seen that APACHE_O is a better test as its ROC curve is closer to that for the perfect test than the one for APACHE II and this is reflected in the larger value for the area under the curve: 0.92 compared to 0.90. Thus APACHE_O could be used instead of APACHE II.

Further details of diagnostic studies, including sample sizes required for comparing alternative diagnostic tests, are given in Machin and Campbell (Chapter 10).[8]

Summary

Correlation:
- Where possible show a scatter diagram of the data.
- In a scatter diagram indicate different categories of observations by using different symbols or colours. For example in Figure 5.3 different symbols were used to indicate the patients' sex.
- The scatter diagram should show all the observations, including coincident data points. Duplicate points can be indicated by a different plotting symbol or an actual number giving the number of coincident points.
- The value of r should be given to two decimal points, together with the P-value if a test of significance is performed.
- The number of observations, n, should be stated.

- If it is necessary to display the correlation between all pairs of a set of three or more variables, this can be done by means of a correlation matrix (Table 5.1) or the preferred graphical equivalent (Figure 5.4).

Regression:
- The equation of the regression line should be given, together with the r^2 value or preferably the residual standard deviation.
- The number of observations, n, used to produce the regression equation should be stated.
- Wherever possible the regression line should be shown in a plot together with the scatter diagram of the raw data with the predictor (explanatory) variable on the X-axis and the dependent variable on the Y-axis. The line should not extent beyond the range of the predictor variable (x).
- The standard error of the slope is useful, as is the P-value from the hypothesis test (for the slope = 0).
- The accuracy used for the coefficients should be related to the accuracy of the raw data. It makes no sense to give an equation that purports to predict birthweight to the nearest 1/100 g when birthweight was actually measured to the nearest grams.
- It is common for the value of the estimate of the intercept to be larger than that of the slope but these are frequently reported to the same number of decimal places. However, when making predictions, it is the slope that is needed with more precision not less, so it should be reported at least as precisely as the intercept.

Method agreement data:
- Report, n, the number of paired observations, for method 1 and method 2.
- A scatter diagram of the measurements of method 1 vs. method 2 with a line of equality ($Y = X$) could be produced.
- Preferably a 'Bland–Altman' style scatter diagram of the difference between the methods on the Y-axis vs. the average of the two methods on the X-axis should be produced.
- The 'Bland–Altman' style scatter diagram should show the line of zero difference alongside the mean difference and the 95% limits of agreement.
- Size of dots should be relative to the number of observations with that combination of values.

ROC curves:
- The number of observations, n, used to produce the ROC curve should be stated.

- The scales for the X (sensitivity) and Y (1 – specificity) axes should range from 0 to 1.
- The line of equality of $y = x$ should be reported.
- The area under the ROC curve should be reported.

References

1 Sivgaru A, Gaines PA, Walters SJ, Beard J, Venables GS. Neuropsychological outcome after carotid angioplasty: randomised controlled trial. The challenge of stroke. *The Lancet conference*. Montreal, Canada: Lancet; 1998.
2 Campbell MJ, Machin D, Walters SJ. *Medical statistics: a textbook for the health sciences*, 4th ed. Chichester: Wiley; 2007.
3 Simpson AG. A comparison of the ability of cranial ultrasound, neonatal neurological assessment and observation of spontaneous movements to predict outcome in preterm infants. Sheffield: University of Sheffield; 2004. PhD thesis.
4 Cleveland WS. Robust locally weighted regression and smoothing scatterplots. *Journal of the American Statistical Association* 1979;**74**:829–36.
5 Hutchinson A, Dean JE, Cooper KL, McIntosh A, Walters SJ, Bath PA, et al. Assessing quality of care from hospital case notes: comparison of two methods. *Quality and Safety in Health Care* 2007.
6 Bland JM, Altman DG. Statistical methods for assessing agreement between two methods of clinical measurement. *The Lancet* 1986;i:307–10.
7 Altman DG. Practical Statistics for Medical Research. London: Chapman & Hall; 1991.
8 Johnson CD, Toh SKC, Campbell MJ. Comparison of APACHE II score and obesity score (APACHE-O) for the prediction of severe acute pancreatitis. *Pancreatology* 2004;**4**:1–6.
9 Machin D, Campbell MJ. *Design of studies for medical research*. Chichester: Wiley; 2005.

Chapter 6 **Data in tables**

6.1 Presenting data and results in tables

Data can be presented in a table as well as or instead of a graph. Although there are no hard and fast rules about when to use a graph and when to use a table, when the results of a study are presented in a report or a paper it is often best to use tables so that the reader can scrutinise the numbers directly. Tables can be useful for displaying information about many variables at once, while graphs can be useful for showing multiple observations on individuals or groups (such as a dotplot or a histogram).

As with graphs, there are a few basic rules of good presentation, including Tufte's golden rule that the amount of information should be maximised for the minimum amount of ink.[1] Tables should be clearly labelled and a brief summary of the contents of a table should always be given in words, either as part of the title or in the main body of the text.

Numerical precision should be consistent throughout and summary statistics such as means and standard deviations (SDs) should not have more than one extra decimal place compared to the raw data. Spurious precision should be avoided, although when certain measures are to be used for further calculations or when presenting the results of analyses greater precision may be necessary.[2]

Solid lines should not be used in the body of a table except to separate labels and summary measures from the main body of the data. However, their use should be kept to a minimum, particularly vertical gridlines, as they can interrupt eye movements, and thus the flow of information.[3] Elsewhere white space can be used to separate data, for example, different variables from each other. Furthermore the information in a table is easier to comprehend if the columns (rather than the rows) contain like information, such as means and SDs, as it is easier to scan down a column than across a row. This may not be possible when there are many variables, such as when presenting the results of a study, but this principle should be followed where possible.

The following sections illustrate the above guidelines and principles for categorical and continuous data.

6.2 Tables for categorical outcome data

Table 3.1 in Chapter 3 described the type of delivery a sample of new mothers experienced when giving birth.[4] Delivery is an example of nominal categorical data (see Figure 1.1) and in this example delivery was classified into six categories. If we were interested in examining whether caesarean section rates differed across hospitals, we could collapse or dichotomise these data into two categories: whether or not the delivery was a caesarean section (planned or emergency). These data are presented in Table 6.1; note that the 12 hospitals have been given fictitious names. The caesarean section rates for each hospital are presented together with the total number of births in that hospital.

Table 6.1 Self-reported caesarean rates (planned or emergency) for 12 maternity hospitals for a 6-week period, $n = 3237$ women[4]

Hospital	Caesarean section rate (%)	(Number of caesarean sections/ total number of births)
King Michael	27.3	(56/205)
Blackwell	25.5	(83/326)
St Stephen's	23.3	(82/352)
Hollyoaks	22.5	(80/356)
The Variance	21.9	(52/237)
Princess Jenny	21.3	(47/221)
Crossroads	20.1	(33/164)
Queen Bess	19.8	(68/344)
Eastend	19.6	(97/495)
The Royal	18.1	(50/277)
Emmerdale	17.7	(23/130)
Coronation	13.1	(17/130)
All hospitals	21.3	(688/3237)

The outcome is presented in the columns and the data for each hospital is reported in the rows. The table conforms to our guidelines for good practice (Box 6.1). The table has a title explaining what is being displayed and the columns and rows are clearly labelled. We have avoided spurious numerical accuracy; the percentages are presented to one decimal place. It is rarely necessary to quote percentages to more than one decimal place. With samples of less than 100 the use of decimal places, when reporting percentages, implies unwarranted precision and should be avoided.[5] In our example, the additional decimal place helps us order the 12 hospitals by their caesarean section rate. Note that these remarks apply only to the presentation of results and rounding should not be used before or during any analysis. While not strictly necessary, enclosing the total number of births in brackets helps distinguish it from the variable of interest: the caesarean rate in each hospital.

The rows (hospitals) have been placed in descending numerical order with the hospital with the largest caesarean rate (King Michael) presented in the first row of the data in the table. Arranged in this way, it is clear from the table that the hospitals with the lowest rates are the hospitals with the fewest births overall. One might conclude that in order to avoid a caesarean section it is good to give birth in a small hospital. However, a more plausible explanation is that women who are in need of a caesarean section or are likely to have complicated labours are more likely to be referred from smaller hospitals to larger, specialist centres.

When the outcome is binary and has only two categories, data for the second category (for the current example: women who did not have a caesarean section) is superfluous and can, as here, be omitted from the table provided that the total number of observations is included. The number of women who did not have a caesarean section can always be calculated as long as the number of observations is reported.

The data in Table 6.1 could also be presented graphically as a bar chart or a stacked bar chart (see Chapter 3 for more details).

6.3 Tables for continuous outcomes

The O'Cathain study also asked about birthweight.[4] Birthweight is an example of continuous data (see Figure 1.1) and in this study it was reported in kilograms (to the nearest 10 g). Table 6.2 reports birthweight by delivery types.

Data on continuous variables, such as birthweight, can be summarised using a measure of central tendency or location along with a measure of spread or variability.[6] If the continuous measurements have a symmetric distribution then the mean and SD are the preferred summary statistics. Alternatively, if the continuous measurements have a skewed distribution (see Chapter 4) then the median and a percentile range, for example, the interquartile range (25th to 75th percentile), are the preferred summary statistics.

In Table 6.2 the rows (delivery type) have been placed in descending numerical order of birthweight, with the heaviest (Forceps delivery) presented

Table 6.2 Self-reported birthweight (kilograms) by delivery type, n = 3178 women[4]

What kind of delivery?	Birthweight (kg)	
	Mean (SD)	n
Forceps delivery	3.46 (0.53)	88
Ventouse (vacuum extractor)	3.44 (0.50)	209
Normal vaginal delivery	3.41 (0.52)	2190
Emergency caesarean section	3.36 (0.70)	426
Planned caesarean section	3.29 (0.59)	249
Vaginal breech delivery	2.81 (0.70)	16
Total	3.39 (0.55)	3178

first. The table has a title explaining what is being displayed and the columns and rows are clearly labelled. As with Table 6.1, the sample size for each delivery type group is reported in the final column of the table as this improves the understanding of data. It is good practice to put the variables of most interest, in this table the mean and SD, in the first data column as they can be immediately read with their associated group label.

In many studies, comparisons are made between different groups. For example, two groups of patients may be given different treatments and the outcomes compared between these treatment groups. Table 6.3 shows an example of a more complex table with three variables: birthweight (the outcome variable in this case); and two categorical variables or factors: parity

Table 6.3 Self-reported birthweight (kg) by delivery type and parity, n = 3176 women[4]

What kind of delivery?	Primiparous birthweight (kg)		Multiparous birthweight (kg)	
	Mean (SD)	n	Mean (SD)	n
Forceps delivery	3.43 (0.54)	75	3.68 (0.44)	13
Emergency caesarean section (once labour had started)	3.40 (0.67)	299	3.27 (0.77)	127
Ventouse (vacuum extractor)	3.37 (0.47)	161	3.66 (0.53)	48
Normal vaginal delivery	3.30 (0.51)	847	3.48 (0.50)	1341
Planned caesarean section	3.15 (0.65)	70	3.35 (0.57)	179
Vaginal breech delivery	3.02 (0.54)	7	2.64 (0.80)	9
Total	3.32 (0.56)	1459	3.45 (0.54)	1717

and delivery type. The outcome, birthweight, is cross classified by parity and delivery type. In this example delivery is ordered by the combined sample size for each delivery type.

6.4 Tables for multiple outcome measures

The use of health-related quality of life (HRQoL) measures is becoming more frequent in clinical trials and health services research, both as primary and secondary outcomes. It is typically assessed by a self-completed questionnaire which asks a series of standardised questions about various aspects or facets of a person's HRQoL. The Medical Outcomes Study 36-Item Short Form (SF-36) is the most commonly used HRQoL measure in the world today.[7,8] It contains 36 questions measuring health across eight dimensions: physical functioning (PF); role limitation because of physical health (RP); social functioning (SF); vitality (VT); bodily pain (BP); mental health (MH); role limitation because of emotional problems (RE) and general health (GH). These eight dimensions are usually regarded as a continuous outcome and are scored on a 0–100 scale, where 100 indicates 'good health'.

Table 6.4 shows SF-36 data from a postal survey of all patients aged 65 years or over registered with 12 general practices. The survey aimed to assess the practicality and validity of using the SF-36 in a community-dwelling population over 65 years old, and obtain population scores in this age group.[9] The table displays summary statistics (mean, SD and sample size) for the eight main dimensions of the SF-36.

The columns contain the ordered age categories and the rows contain the eight SF-36 dimensions. The column variable, age, has a natural ordering so the columns are clearly ordered by the age categories: the row variables (the eight SF-36 dimensions) have no natural ordering, in this example they are ordered by the dimension with the highest overall mean score (social function). The footnote to the table also explains how the SF-36 is scaled. The units and scale of HRQoL may be unfamiliar to many readers (unlike other outcomes such as birthweight) and the footnote helps in the understanding and interpretation of the mean SF-36 dimension scores. Most HRQoL measures generate a scale or scores that have no natural units and have varying scale ranges: for some a high score implies good HRQoL and for others a high score implies poor HRQoL. With outcomes with unfamiliar scales or units of measurement it is recommended to add a footnote to tables, explaining the scale of measurement to help interpretation of the data presented.

The table has a title explaining what is being displayed and the columns and rows are clearly labelled. Enclosing the SDs in brackets helps distinguish the variability in the HRQoL data from the mean dimension score.

Table 6.4 Mean (SD) scores and samples sizes, for the eight dimensions of the SF-36* by age, $n = 5841$[9]

		Age (years)					
		65–69	70–74	75–79	80–84	85+	Group total
Social function	Mean	78.2	75.1	69.6	61.0	48.9	70.9
	SD	(28.4)	(29.8)	(31.1)	(33.1)	(32.8)	(31.5)
	n	1641	1720	1274	746	460	5841
Mental health	Mean	72.2	71.7	70.4	67.8	65.9	70.6
	SD	(20.3)	(19.8)	(19.5)	(20.2)	(21.1)	(20.1)
	n	1641	1720	1274	746	460	5841
Bodily pain	Mean	66.4	63.2	61.5	55.3	53.4	62.0
	SD	(27.7)	(27.8)	(28.5)	(28.6)	(29.4)	(28.5)
	n	1641	1720	1274	746	460	5841
Role emotional	Mean	65.8	60.0	52.8	45.5	42.8	56.9
	SD	(42.4)	(43.8)	(44.7)	(44.3)	(45.8)	(44.5)
	n	1641	1720	1274	746	460	5841
Physical function	Mean	65.4	59.5	52.6	42.0	27.6	54.9
	SD	(28.9)	(29.7)	(29.7)	(30.0)	(26.4)	(31.2)
	n	1641	1720	1274	746	460	5841
General health	Mean	57.8	56.6	54.7	49.5	46.5	54.8
	SD	(24.1)	(23.6)	(22.9)	(23.2)	(21.4)	(23.6)
	n	1641	1720	1274	746	460	5841
Vitality	Mean	56.6	53.8	50.6	44.7	39.0	51.5
	SD	(23.1)	(22.5)	(21.9)	(22.7)	(21.7)	(23.1)
	n	1641	1720	1274	746	460	5841
Role physical	Mean	55.6	46.8	41.2	30.2	25.2	44.2
	SD	(42.7)	(43.0)	(41.8)	(38.4)	(35.8)	(42.6)
	n	1641	1720	1274	746	460	5841

* The dimensions of the SF-36 are scored on a 0 (worst possible health) to 100 (best possible health) scale.

The sample size for each age group is reported underneath the SD. As the SF-36 dimensions are scored on a 0–100 scale, the means and SDs for the various dimensions are reported to one decimal place in the table to avoid the spurious numerical precision discussed earlier.

Summary

• The amount of information should be maximised for the minimum amount of ink.

- Numerical precision should be consistent throughout a paper or presentation, as far as possible.
- Avoid spurious accuracy. Bear in mind the precision of the original data. Numbers should be rounded to two effective digits.
- The number of observations on which the data being presented is based should always be displayed.
- Quantitative data should be summarised using either the mean and SD (for symmetrically distributed data) or the median and IQR or range (for skewed data). The number of observations on which these summary measures are based should be included for each result in the table.
- Categorical data should be summarised as frequencies and percentages. As with quantitative data, the number of observations should be included.
- Tables should have a title explaining what is being displayed and columns and rows should be clearly labelled.
- Solid lines in tables should be kept to a minimum.
- Rows and columns should be ordered by size (if there is no natural ordering).

References

1 Tufte ER. *The visual display of quantitative information*. Cheshire, Connecticut: Graphics Press; 1983.
2 Altman DG, Bland JM. Presentation of numerical data. *British Medical Journal* 1996;**312**:572.
3. Ehrenberg A.S.C. A primer in data reduction. Chichester. John Wiley & Sons Ltd; 1982.
4 O'Cathain A, Walters S, Nicholl JP, Thomas KJ, Kirkham M. Use of evidence based leaflets to promote informed choice in maternity care: randomised controlled trial in everyday practice. *British Medical Journal* 2002;**324**:643–6.
5 Altman DG, Machin D, Bryant T, Gardner MJ. *Statistics with confidence*, 2nd ed. London: BMJ Books; 2000.
6 Campbell MJ, Machin D, Walters SJ. *Medical statistics: a textbook for the health sciences*, 4th ed. Chichester: Wiley; 2007.
7 Brazier JE, Harper R, Jones NMB, O'Cathain A, Thomas KJ, Usherwood T, et al. Validating the SF-36 health survey questionnaire: new outcome measure for primary care. *British Medical Journal* 1992;**305**:160–4.
8 Ware JE, Snow KK, Kosinski M, Gandek B. *SF-36 Health survey manual and interpretation guide*. Boston: The Health Institute, New England Medical Centre; 1993.
9 Walters SJ, Munro JF, Brazier JE. Using the SF-36 with older adults: a cross-sectional community-based survey. *Age and Ageing* 2001;**30**:337–43.

Chapter 7 **Reporting study results**

7.1 Introduction

In many studies comparisons are made between different groups. For example, in a randomised controlled trial (RCT), two groups of patients may be randomly allocated to different treatments and the outcomes for these different groups are subsequently compared. This chapter will describe ways of tabulating and displaying outcome data when we are interested in comparing two groups; both for a RCT and more generally for studies that involve any comparison between two groups. However, it is worth noting that the information presented in this chapter can be generalised to more than two groups.

The first part of this chapter will deal with how to display different types of outcome data, including the results of logistic and multiple regression analyses. In addition, further issues particular to the reporting of RCTs will be covered, as will methods for displaying the results of meta-analyses. This chapter will focus on the type of information and statistics that should be displayed for study outcomes. Good practice with respect to displaying data in tables will only be mentioned briefly, as this has been covered elsewhere in the book (Chapter 6).

7.2 Tabulating categorical outcomes

The simplest study outcomes are binary categorical outcomes, that is, those with only two categories, for example dead or alive, cured or not cured. One of the main outcomes from the leg ulcer trial described earlier (Chap 1) was whether the leg ulcer had healed or not after 3 months of treatment and follow-up.[1]

With two independent groups (intervention or control) and a binary categorical outcome (healed or not healed), one way of displaying these data is to cross-tabulate them as shown in Table 7.1. This is an example of a 2-by-2 contingency table with 2 rows for treatment and 2 columns for outcome, and it is said to have four cells (2 × 2) (see also Chapter 3). The most appropriate comparative summary measure for these data is the difference in proportions healed between the two groups.

The important contrast is between the 20% healed in the intervention group compared to 16% in the control group. Since English script reads naturally from left to right, it is recommended that the data for treatment groups is in the columns in order that differences between groups can be compared side by side as shown in Table 7.1.

Another advantage of the format in Table 7.1 is that with several outcomes we can place the data for the different outcomes underneath each other in separate rows. For example, Table 7.2 shows the ulcer healing rates at 3 and 12 months. This format, with the groups in the columns, is also

Table 7.1 Cross-tabulation of treatment group (in columns) vs. outcome (in rows) ulcer healed or not healed at 12 weeks (n = 206)[1]

	Group	
	Intervention % (n = 106)	Control % (n = 100)
Outcome		
Healed	20% (21)	16% (16)
Not healed	80% (85)	84% (84)

Table 7.2 Ulcer healing rates at 3 and 12 months follow-up by treatment group (maximum n = 206)[1]

	Group		Difference in percentages[a] (95% CI)	P-value[b]	Relaive Risk[c] (95% CI)
	Intervention	Control			
Outcome					
Healed at 3 months	20% (21/106)	16% (16/100)	4% (−7 to 14)	0.47	1.25 (0.69–2.23)
Healed at 12 months	52% (42/81)	42% (33/79)	10% (−5 to 25)	0.20	1.24 (0.89–1.73)

CI: Confidence interval.
[a]A positive difference indicates that the intervention group does better than the control group.
[b]P-values from chi-squared test.
[c]A relative risk > 1 indicates that the intervention group does better than the control group.

favoured by leading medical journals, such as the *British Medical Journal*. Note that no decimal places are reported for the percentages of ulcers healed or the difference, which makes the table clearer. The denominator is presented for all the outcomes and thus it is clear that the sample size is lower for the 12-month comparison. Also presented is a column with the absolute difference in ulcer healing rates between the two groups, its 95% confidence interval and the *P*-value associated with this comparison. It is recommended that when presenting confidence intervals the word 'to' is used to link the lower and upper limits rather than a dash symbol '–' as it can sometimes be difficult to know whether the upper limit is negative or not if the dash symbol is used. When presenting a *P*-value it is important to make clear what statistical test was used to derive it. In Table 7.2 the *P*-value has come from the chi-squared test.

For two groups with a binary outcome there are several other ways of comparing the groups, not just a comparison of two proportions. Alternatives include: the relative risk (RR); odds ratio (OR) and number needed to treat (NNT). See Campbell et al. (2007) for more details on how to calculate these summary measures.[2] The last column of data in Table 7.2 shows the RR of an ulcer healing in the intervention group compared to an ulcer healing in the control group, together with its 95% confidence interval.

When there are more than two categories for the outcome variable, such as a five point symptom score scale (much better, better, same, worse, much worse), these may also be incorporated in a format similar to Table 7.2, with a separate line for each category of the variable. If the categories have a natural ordering such as the pain scale above, then this ordering should be preserved. If however, there is no natural ordering then the categories should be ordered by size.

7.3 Tabulating the results of logistic regression analysis

The previous section in this chapter described a method for displaying categorical outcome data. In addition to the grouping variable it is often important to adjust for other explanatory variables, in which case a logistic regression is usually carried out. One of the outcomes from the leg ulcer study was ulcer status at 12 weeks (healed/not healed) and the results of a logistic regression to assess the impact of various explanatory variables on ulcer state at 12 weeks is presented in Table 7.3. When reporting the results of a logistic regression analysis, as a minimum the estimated OR for the regression coefficients, their confidence intervals and associated *P*-values should be presented. The sample size that the regression was based upon should also be reported. If space allows, the regression coefficient and its

Table 7.3 Estimated OR from the multiple logistic regression model to predict ulcer status (healed or not healed) at 12 weeks from baseline ulcer area, gender, marital status and treatment group in 187 patients with venous leg ulcers[1]

	OR (95% CI)	P-value
Intercept	0.15	0.003
Baseline ulcer area (cm^2)	0.89 (0.82 to 0.96)	0.004
Gender (0 = male, 1 = female)	3.37 (1.21 to 9.34)	0.020
Marital status		0.670
Married (reference category)	1.00	
Single (relative to married)	1.83 (0.47 to 7.19)	0.384
Divorced (relative to married)	0.49 (0.05 to 4.81)	0.543
Widowed (relative to married)	0.84 (0.35 to 2.00)	0.695
Group (0 = Control, 1 = Intervention)	1.80 (0.79 to 4.09)	0.159

CI: Confidence interval.
Hosmer and Lemeshow test, $\chi^2 = 11.22$ on 8 degrees of freedom, $P = 0.19$.
Y variable: Ulcer healed at 12 weeks (0 = No, 1 = Yes).

standard error (SE) can also be reported, but as this is on a logarithmic scale, it is not as helpful as the estimated OR. For logistic regression it is also helpful to give some information about the goodness of fit of the model to the data. The simplest statistic for doing this is the Hosmer and Lemeshow chi-squared statistics and we would recommend this is reported together with the degrees of freedom and *P*-value so that the reader can judge whether or not the model adequately fits the data.[3]

7.4 Tabulating quantitative outcomes

In addition to displaying categorical outcomes, outcome data may be quantitative, either count or continuous. As part of a RCT comparing traditional acupuncture with usual care for non-specific low back pain, HRQoL was measured at 12 months, using the SF-36.[4] These data are shown in Table 7.4. Data for the two treatment groups is arranged in the columns and the rows correspond to the eight SF-36 dimensions, and are ordered by mean difference. The mean dimension scores (and their variability) are described separately for each group. A 95% confidence interval for the treatment effect, (difference in mean scores), is reported. Exact *P*-values are reported to two significant figures in the last column of the table. A footnote to the table is included describing how the SF-36 is scaled and scored, what hypothesis test has been performed and how the treatment effect (mean difference) should be interpreted. Since the SF-36 is scored on a 0–100 scale

Table 7.4 Mean SF-36 dimension scores at 12 months by treatment group[4]

SF-36 dimension[a]	Treatment group				Mean difference[b] (95% CI)	P-value[c]
	Usual care		Acupuncture			
	n	Mean (SD)	n	Mean (SD)		
Pain	68	58.3 (22.2)	147	64.0 (25.6)	5.7 (−1.4 to 12.8)	0.12
Role-physical	57	61.8 (42.8)	134	66.0 (40.0)	4.2 (−8.5 to 17.0)	0.52
Role-emotional	57	78.4 (35.9)	133	78.2 (35.3)	−0.2 (−11.2 to 10.9)	0.98
General health	56	65.4 (19.3)	134	64.8 (21.8)	−0.6 (−7.2 to 6.1)	0.87
Physical functioning	57	73.4 (20.9)	133	71.7 (25.8)	−1.7 (−9.4 to 5.9)	0.65
Vitality	56	57.0 (21.6)	135	54.1 (23.3)	−2.9 (−10.0 to 4.3)	0.43
Social functioning	68	80.7 (22.1)	147	77.8 (25.2)	−2.9 (−10.0 to 4.1)	0.41
Mental health	56	73.3 (15.4)	135	69.0 (20.4)	−4.3 (−10.3 to 1.6)	0.15

CI: Confidence interval.
[a]The SF-36 dimensions are scored on a 0 (poor) to 100 (good health) scale.
[b]A positive mean difference indicates the acupuncture group has the better HRQoL.
[c]P-value from two independent samples t-test.

these data are reported to a precision of one decimal place. Note that as the number of observations varies considerably across the eight dimensions a second table could also be produced for those individuals who had data on all dimensions.

7.5 Plots for displaying outcome data

A useful plot for displaying continuous outcome data, when there are multiple variables all measured on the same scale, such as for the HRQoL data in Table 7.4 is the *spider or radar plot*. Figure 7.1 shows a radar plot for the mean SF-36 dimension scores, at 12 months follow-up, by treatment group for the data presented in Table 7.4. The radar plot has eight spokes corresponding to the eight dimensions of the SF-36, with the centre point of the plot indicating a score of 0. It is clear from this plot that the two treatments groups have similar mean HRQoL for all eight dimensions of the SF-36, although Figure 7.1 conceals the fact that the sample size for each dimension varies considerably. We could report the number of subjects for each outcome, but this would make the chart look rather messy. An alternative strategy would be redraw the plot but including only those subjects who had data for all outcomes.

The radar plot of Figure 7.1 clearly displays the mean SF-36 dimension scores by treatment group. However, for comparison purposes, what is required is the contrast or difference in outcomes between the groups and the associated uncertainty or confidence interval around this estimated treatment effect. These can be shown graphically using a forest plot similar to those used for displaying the results of meta-analyses and systematic reviews, described later in this chapter. Figure 7.2 shows a forest plot of the estimated treatment effect (mean difference in SF-36 scores between the acupuncture and usual care groups) and the corresponding confidence interval, at 12 months, for the eight dimensions of the SF-36.[4]

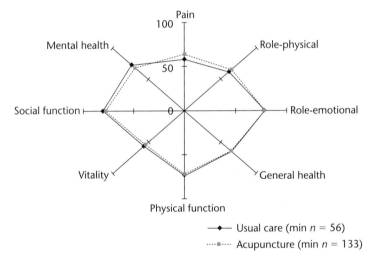

Figure 7.1 Radar or spider plot with mean scores, at 12 months follow-up, for the eight dimensions of the SF-36 by treatment group, Note that the SF-36 dimensions are scored on a 0 (poor) to 100 (good) health scale.[4]

Figure 7.2 is visually impressive and the lack of any treatment effect for HRQoL is readily apparent. Also note that the numbers used for each comparison are clearly displayed. This chart can be particularly useful in conference presentations when much information needs to be conveyed to the audience in a limited amount of time. However, much of the data presented

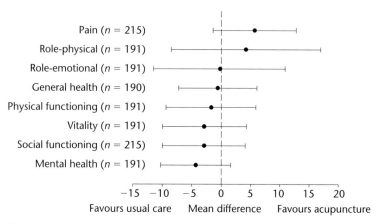

Figure 7.2 Estimated treatment effect (mean difference in SF-36 score between the acupuncture and usual care groups) and the corresponding 95% confidence interval, at 12 months, for the eight dimensions of the SF-36.[4]

in Table 7.4 are not shown. For example the sample size per treatment group and mean scores (and their variability) are omitted. These are important results and this information should be reported. Hence for presentation in a scientific report or paper, Table 7.4 is preferred.

Forest plots can also be useful when reporting the results of equivalence trials as the limits of equivalence can be easily included on the chart. The objective of an equivalence trial is to show that a new therapy has the same (or very similar) effect as an existing therapy, with regards to the outcome of interest. Before an equivalence trial is carried out the limits of equivalence are agreed, so that after the trial a decision can be made as to whether the treatments are equivalent. These pre-specified limits should be narrow enough to exclude any difference of clinical importance. After the trial, equivalence is usually accepted if the confidence interval for any observed treatment difference is within the limits of equivalence and includes a value of zero difference.

Bowns et al. report the results of a RCT of telemedicine in dermatology.[5] The objectives of this study were to compare the clinical equivalence of store-and-forward teledermatology (intervention) with conventional face-to-face consultation (control) in setting a management plan for new adult outpatient referrals. A total of 208 patients were randomised (111 in the telemedicine group and 97 in the control group) and 165 patients (92 intervention, 73 control) had data for analysis.

For both the teledermatology and conventional consultation groups, the diagnosis and management of each case was examined by an independent consultant. The main outcome measure was the agreement between the consultant who had managed the case and the independent consultant, on the initial diagnosis and management of the patient. It was decided that the two methods (teledermatology and conventional consultation) would be regarded as diagnostically equivalent if the 95% confidence limits for the difference in proportions (the proportions in the two groups, respectively, agreeing with the independent opinion) lay wholly within the interval −0.1 to 0.1, the range of clinical equivalence.

The results for different outcomes from this trial are displayed as a forest plot in Figure 7.3, which also includes the limits of equivalence. It is immediately clear from this plot that the two treatments could not be regarded as equivalent since the lower limits of the confidence interval estimates for all four outcomes are outside the pre-specified range of clinical equivalence.

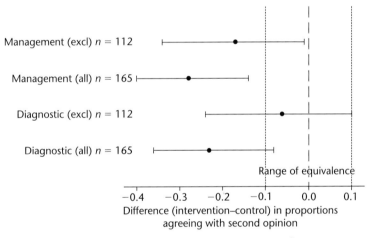

Figure 7.3 Equivalence of diagnostic and management outcomes.[5]
Excl: Excluding patients whose management was transferred.

7.6 Tabulating the results of regression analyses

While Table 7.4 shows the result of a simple comparison between two groups, there are usually several explanatory variables that are of interest. It is common to investigate these variables using a technique known as multiple regression analysis. This allows for the influence of several explanatory variables on the outcome of interest to be investigated simultaneously. For example, in the Simpson study of pre-term babies, described in Chapter 5, other variables apart from gestation, such as maternal age and the baby's gender, may have a role to play in determining birthweight and these can be included in the regression model to examine what their influence on birthweight is, over and above that exerted by gestation.[6]

With two or more explanatory variables in the regression model it is not possible in a single two-dimensional graph to produce a scatter plot of the *Y*-variable against all the *X*-variables simultaneously. In these circumstances we can display the matrix of scatter diagrams showing each of the two-way relationships between the dependent and explanatory variables, such as Figure 5.4.

However, it is possible to show the relationship between birthweight and all the explanatory variables in a table. When tabulating the results of a regression analysis, as a minimum, it is important to display the estimated regression coefficients, *b*, and their associated confidence intervals and *P*-values, as illustrated in Table 7.5. It can also be helpful if the SEs of the coefficients are included. Note that as males are coded 0 and females are coded 1, the negative sign attached to the coefficient for gender indicates that girls are on average 0.1 kg lighter than boys. For the continuous explanatory variables the regression coefficients indicate the effect on the outcome variable (in this case birthweight) of a unit change in the value of the continuous variable. As well as the information outlined above, it is also important to include the value of the R^2 statistic as this is indicative of how well the fitted model describes the data. In this case, the R^2 value of 0.68 suggests that a multiple regression model, containing gender, gestation and maternal age as predictors, explains 68% of the variability in the outcome birthweight. Although space will not always allow, if possible it is good practice to include the SE of the coefficient and the associated *t* statistic for the individual *P*-values. While rarely done, it can also be helpful to include the residual standard deviation (SD) so that the prediction error, *s*, can be calculated.

Table 7.5 Estimated coefficients from the multiple regression model to predict birthweight from gender, gestation and maternal age in 98 pre-term babies[6]

	Coefficient (SE)	95% CI	P-value
Intercept	−2.56 (0.31)	−3.18 to −1.93	<0.001
Gender (0 = male, 1 = female)	−0.11 (0.05)	−0.20 to −0.006	0.04
Gestation (weeks)	0.13 (0.01)	0.11 to 0.15	0.001
Maternal age (years)	0.001 (0.004)	−0.007 to 0.009	0.82

CI: Confidence interval.
Y or dependent variable: birthweight (kg).
$R^2 = 0.68$.
Residual SD = 0.244 kg.

If we suspect that observed differences, or imbalance, between the groups at the start of the study may have affected the outcome we can use multiple regression analysis to adjust for these.[2] In this case we are rarely interested in estimating the effect of these baseline differences. Thus we do not necessarily wish to report the regression coefficients for these covariates, but we want to ensure that any estimates of the differences between groups that are produced have taken account of them. Table 7.6 shows the recommended way of tabulating outcomes after adjusting for other (nuisance) variables. The unadjusted treatment effect (with its confidence interval) should be presented alongside the adjusted treatment effect (with its confidence interval). The P-values from the two hypothesis tests can also be reported, although this is not essential. The footnote makes clear what covariates have been used to adjust the treatment comparison between the groups – again this information should be made clear either in the table or the title. In this example the outcome, 12 month SF-36 pain score, was adjusted for baseline pain score and four other baseline covariates: duration of current episode of pain (in weeks), expectation of back pain in 6 months, SF-36 physical functioning and reported pain in legs.

It is important to make clear the sample size for both the unadjusted and adjusted analysis. Ideally they should both contain the same number of subjects. However, frequently some of the covariates used in the adjusted analysis are missing for one or two patients, even though the main outcome for these patients was recorded. Table 7.6 shows that 215 (147 acupuncture: 68 usual care) patients had a valid SF-36 pain score at both baseline and 12

Table 7.6 Unadjusted and adjusted differences in SF-36 pain outcome scores between acupuncture and usual care groups at 12 months[4]

SF-36 dimension[a]	Treatment group				Unadjusted[b] Difference[c] (95% CI)	P-value	Adjusted[b] Difference[c] (95% CI)	P-value
	Usual care		Acupuncture					
	n	Mean (SD)	n	Mean (SD)				
Pain	68	58.3 (22.2)	147	64.0 (25.6)	5.7 (−1.4 to 12.8)	0.12	6.0 (−0.6 to 12.6)	0.07

CI: Confidence interval.
[a]The SF-36 pain dimension is scored on a 0–100 (no pain) scale.
[b]n = 212 difference adjusted for baseline pain score and other baseline covariates: duration of current episode of pain (in weeks), expectation of back pain in 6 months, SF-36 physical functioning and reported pain in legs.
[c]Improvement is indicated by a positive difference on the SF-36 pain dimension.

months follow-up. For the adjusted analysis, three patients did not have one or more of the covariates recorded at baseline, so they are excluded from this analysis. In this example, it is unlikely that excluding three patients from the adjusted analysis will affect the comparisons between the unadjusted and adjusted treatment effects.

7.7 Reporting results for repeated measures data

In many studies it is common for there to be several follow-up assessments, resulting in repeated measures data. For example, RCTs are by their definition prospective longitudinal studies. Patients are randomly allocated to different treatments and followed over time and patients are often measured at several time points.

Repeated measurements data must be analyzed carefully and this should be reflected in the methods chosen to display them. A series of hypothesis tests comparing the groups at each follow-up time point is not recommended, although this is often found in the medical literature. The data must be either modelled properly[7] or the repeated assessments can be aggregated into a single summary measure (such as the area under the curve (AUC)) and this can then be compared between groups.[8] As part of the acupuncture trial, the patients' HRQoL was assessed at baseline (0), 3, 12 and 24 months using the SF-36.[4] Table 7.7 shows one way of presenting such data for the pain dimension of the SF-36.

In Table 7.7 the SF-36 pain scores are not tested at each time point. The results of hypothesis tests and confidence intervals are only presented for the two summary measures in the last two rows of the table, mean follow-up pain score and pain AUC. The sample size at each of the follow-up time points varies and therefore it is important to report the sample size for each row of the data. If the sample size varies considerably across assessment times Table 7.7 can be redrawn for only those patients who completed all four assessments. This makes it easier to see how the mean pain scores vary over time for the same patients.

The data in Table 7.7 can be plotted as a line graph (Figure 7.4), with a separate line for each group. Figure 7.4 clearly shows how the pain outcome varies both over time and between groups. The groups have similar mean pain scores at baseline and 3 months, but by 12 and 24 months follow-up the mean scores have started to diverge with the acupuncture group having the better outcome. If the sample size varies across time it is important that the time points are not joined using solid lines, since we are not measuring the same people at each time point. If the plot had been only for those individuals who had data at each time point it would be legitimate to join

Table 7.7 Mean SF-36 pain scores over time by treatment group with all valid patients at each time point[4]

SF-36 dimension[a]	Usual care		Acupuncture		Mean difference[b] (95% CI)	P-value[c]
	n	Mean (SD)	n	Mean (SD)		
0 m – SF-36 pain	80	30.4 (18.0)	159	30.8 (16.2)		
3 m – SF-36 pain	71	55.4 (25.4)	146	60.9 (23.0)		
12 m – SF-36 pain	68	58.3 (22.2)	147	64.0 (25.6)		
24 m – SF-36 pain	59	59.5 (23.4)	123	67.8 (24.1)		
Mean follow-up SF-36 pain score	76	57.2 (19.8)	153	63.4 (20.9)	6.3 (0.6–12.0)	0.03
Pain AUC	55	127.1 (41.7)	118	141.1 (44.6)	14.0 (−0.1 to 28.1)	0.05

CI: Confidence interval.
[a]The SF-36 pain dimension is scored on a 0 (alot) to 100 (no) pain scale.
[b]A positive mean difference indicates the acupuncture group has the better HRQoL.
[c]P-value from two independent samples t-test.

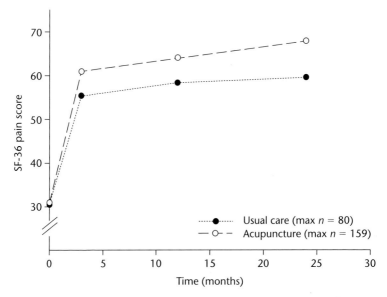

Figure 7.4 Profile of mean SF-36 pain scores over time by treatment group.[4]

the mean pain scores together with solid lines. One other important feature of this graph is the exclusion of confidence intervals for the means at each time period. To do so would be to imply that it is appropriate to compare the groups at each time point. As it is inappropriate to perform a significance test at each time period, so it is inappropriate to include confidence intervals for the estimates of the mean at each time point.

7.8 Randomised controlled trials

It is important that RCTs are reported adequately, since they have considerable potential to affect patient care. Concern over the variability in the quality of the reporting of RCTs in the medical literature lead to the development of the Consolidation of Standards for Reporting Trials (CONSORT) statement.[9] It consists of a flow diagram and a checklist of 22 items which should be reported in the paper for every RCT (see Table A7.1 in the appendix). While the CONSORT statement was designed to be used to report the results of RCTs, only 5 of the 22 items in the checklist specifically apply to RCTs and the majority of the items are applicable for most other studies that collect quantitative data. Therefore we recommend that the flow diagram and CONSORT checklist be used as a guideline for the reporting of the results of other studies including cross-sectional surveys and other observational studies. More details can be found at http://www.consort-statement.org.

7.9 Patient flow diagram

Figure 7.5 shows a *CONSORT flow diagram* for the acupuncture trial.[4] It allows readers to understand quickly how many eligible participants were randomly assigned to each arm of the trial and whether there are any imbalances with respect to the numbers of patients withdrawing from or failing to comply with their assigned treatment. The group allocation was on a 2:1 basis in favour of acupuncture and from Figure 7.5 it is easy to see that of the 241 eligible patients consented to be randomised, 160 patients were offered acupuncture and 81 were allocated to usual care. One patient in each group withdrew from the study immediately after randomisation. Ideally the reasons for patients dropping out should be recorded. At 12 months follow-up there were 215 patients with outcome data available for analysis (147 in the acupuncture group and 68 in the usual care group). By 24 months follow-up the number of patients with data available for analysis had dropped further to 182.

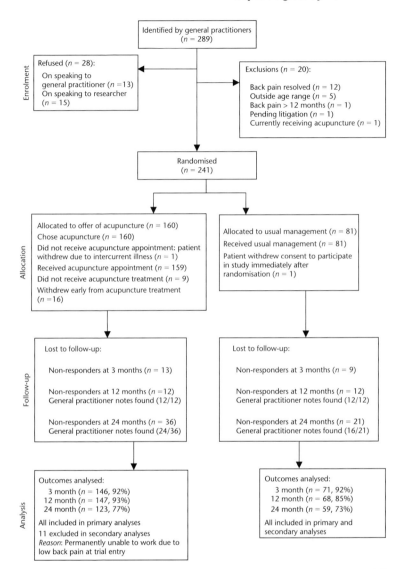

Figure 7.5 Patient progress through trial: CONSORT flow chart for acupuncture study.[4]

7.10 Comparison of entry characteristics

The first table in the report of a RCT should provide a summary of the entry or baseline characteristics of the patients in the study groups. It is important to show that the groups are similar with respect to variables that

Table 7.8 Baseline characteristics of patients by treatment group[4]

Characteristic		Treatment group			
		Usual care		Acupuncture	
		n	Mean or %	*n*	Mean or %
Age (years)		80	44.0	159	41.9
(range)			(20–64)		(26–64)
Duration of back		80	16.7	159	17.1
pain (weeks) (SD)			(14.6)		(13.5)
SF-36 pain (SD)		80	30.4	159	30.8
			(18.0)		(16.2)
Gender	Male	34/80	(43)	60/159	(38)
Number of previous	None	13	(16)	25	(16)
episodes of low	1–5	23	(29)	57	(36)
back pain	>5	44	(55)	77	(48)
Expectation of back	Better	30	(38)	80	(51)
pain in 6 months	Same	37	(46)	56	(35)
	Worse	12	(16)	21	(13)

may have an impact on the patient's response,[10] although performing a hypothesis test to compare the baseline characteristics of the groups is not recommended. If the randomisation has been performed properly, any differences between the two treatment groups must be due to chance.

The table of baseline characteristics, such as Table 7.8 for the acupuncture trial allows the reader to see if there are any variables with known or suspected prognostic importance that are not closely balanced between the groups. Data for the intervention and control groups are reported in columns and the baseline variables are reported by row. For the categorical outcomes the percentages are also reported; this helps compare the two groups, since the 2:1 randomisation schedule has resulted in twice as many patients in the acupuncture arm of the trial. For outcomes with only two categories the result should be given as x/n (y%). For more than two categories the total should be given as a separate row to avoid repeating it for each category and to enable a check that all categories are present. In this way we can see there is one missing value in 'expectation of back pain' in the control group and two missing values in the intervention group.

From the CONSORT flow diagram in Figure 7.5 we see that 241 patients were randomised in the acupuncture study but only 182 (i.e. 75% of the original cohort) had outcomes at 24 months that were analysable. In the

Table 7.9 Baseline characteristics of patients of all recruited patients ($n = 239$) vs. those with outcomes for analysis at 24 months ($n = 182$) by group[4]

Characteristic		Treatment group						
		Usual care				Acupuncture		
		All patients ($n = 80$)		Analysed at 24 months ($n = 59$)		All patients ($n = 159$)		Analysed at 24 months ($n = 123$)
		n	Mean	n	Mean	n	Mean	n	Mean
Age (years) (range)		80	44.0 (20–64)	59	45.5 (20–64)	159	41.9 (26–64)	123	42.5 (26–64)
Duration of back pain (weeks) (SD)		80	16.7 (14.6)	59	16.0 (14.1)	159	17.1 (13.5)	123	17.0 (13.3)
SF-36 pain (SD)		80	30.4 (18.0)	59	29.9 (18.7)	159	30.8 (16.2)	123	30.8 (16.6)
Gender	Male	34	(43%)	23	(39%)	60	(38%)	44	(36%)
Number of previous episodes of low back pain	None	13	(16%)	10	(17%)	25	(16%)	20	(16%)
	1–5	23	(29%)	16	(27%)	57	(36%)	42	(34%)
	>5	44	(55%)	33	(56%)	77	(48%)	61	(50%)
Expectation of back pain in 6 months	Better	30	(38%)	25	(42%)	80	(51%)	57	(47%)
	Same	37	(46%)	23	(39%)	56	(35%)	47	(39%)
	Worse	12	(16%)	10	(17%)	21	(13%)	17	(14%)
	Don't know	1	(1%)	1	(2%)	1	(1%)	1	(1%)

original cohort of 239 patients Table 7.8 clearly shows that the two groups were well matched at baseline. However, withdrawal may be caused by treatment-related side effects. Whatever the reason, the incomplete data may compromise the initial baseline balance between the two treatment groups. Thus a table comparing the baseline characteristics of those randomised with those actually analysed is also useful, though rarely reported (Table 7.9).

7.11 Forest plots

A forest plot is commonly used for displaying the quantitative results of studies included in meta-analyses and systematic reviews. The forest plot consists of a graph that shows the estimated effect and the corresponding

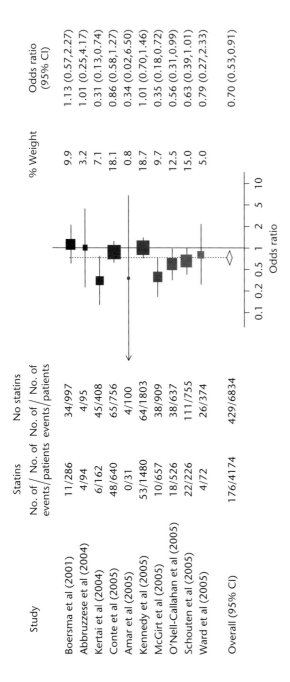

Figure 7.6 Forest plot of OR of death or acute coronary syndrome (for statins vs. no statins) in 10 non-cardiac surgery studies investigating the use of statins during the perioperative period to reduce the risk of cardiovascular events.[11]

Study	Statins No. of / No. of events/patients	No statins No. of / No. of events/patients	% Weight	Odds ratio (95% CI)
Boersma et al (2001)	11/286	34/997	9.9	1.13 (0.57,2.27)
Abbruzzese et al (2004)	4/94	4/95	3.2	1.01 (0.25,4.17)
Kertai et al (2004)	6/162	45/408	7.1	0.31 (0.13,0.74)
Conte et al (2005)	48/640	65/756	18.1	0.86 (0.58,1.27)
Amar et al (2005)	0/31	4/100	0.8	0.34 (0.02,6.50)
Kennedy et al (2005)	53/1480	64/1803	18.7	1.01 (0.70,1.46)
McGirt et al (2005)	10/657	38/909	9.7	0.35 (0.18,0.72)
O'Nell-Callahan et al (2005)	18/526	38/637	12.5	0.56 (0.31,0.99)
Schouten et al (2005)	22/226	111/755	15.0	0.63 (0.39,1.01)
Ward et al (2005)	4/72	26/374	5.0	0.79 (0.27,2.33)
Overall (95% CI)	176/4174	429/6834		0.70 (0.53,0.91)

confidence interval from each study. The forest plot can also be used for displaying the results of different outcomes within the same study, provided that they are measured on the same scale (see Figures 7.2 and 7.3). Figure 7.6 is an example of a forest plot from a meta-analysis of 10 non-cardiac surgery studies investigating the use of statins during the perioperative period to reduce the risk of cardiovascular events.[11] The outcome for each study was the OR of death or acute coronary syndrome for statins vs. no statins.

Figure 7.6 contains both graphical and tabular elements. Data from each study are summarised in horizontal rows, with the name of the study's first author, the year of publication, summary measure of the treatment effect and confidence interval and the percentage weight each study is given in the overall meta-analysis. The estimates of the treatment effect are marked by squares and the associated uncertainty shown by horizontal lines extending between the upper and lower confidence intervals. The size of the block varies between studies to reflect the weight given to each in the meta-analysis, more influential studies having the larger blocks. In addition this counters a tendency for the viewer's eyes to be drawn to the studies which have the widest confidence interval estimates, and are therefore graphically more impressive (but are the least significant).[12] Sometimes, too, the individual lines are ordered by date of study (as here), by some index of study quality or by the point estimate of effect size.

The overall estimate of effect from all the studies combined is marked at the bottom of the plot as a diamond, the central points indicating the point estimate while the outer points mark the confidence limits. A vertical line is drawn on the chart at the meta-analytical point estimate. From the plots it is often possible to assess visually the degree of heterogeneity in study results by noting the overlap of confidence intervals of individual studies with the overall combined point estimate from the meta-analysis.

7.12 Funnel plots

Funnel plots are a particular type of scatter plot used to detect publication bias in meta-analyses and systematic reviews.[13] For each study in a review the estimated treatment effect is plotted against a measure of trial precision such as the variance or SE of the treatment effect, or study sample size (Figure 7.7). In a change from the standard graphical practice for scatter plots where the outcome variable or treatment effect is plotted on the vertical axis (see Chapter 5), funnel plots depict precision (variance of the treatment effect or sample size) on the vertical axis and the treatment effect on the horizontal axis. The overall combined summary from the meta-analysis may be marked by a vertical line.

84 **How to Display Data**

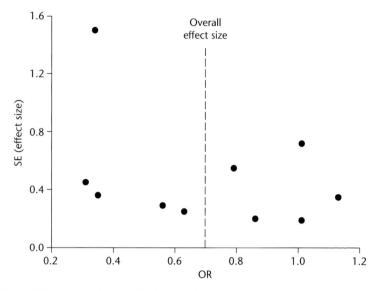

Figure 7.7 Funnel plot of SE of the treatment effect against OR of death or acute coronary syndrome (for statins vs. no statins) in 10 non-cardiac surgery studies investigating the use of statins during the perioperative period to reduce the risk of cardiovascular events, with the overall effect size (OR of 0.70).[11]

When all study results are published it is expected that the studies will have a symmetrical distribution around the average or overall effect line, the spread of studies with low precision being larger than that of studies with high precision, resulting in a funnel-like shape. Some graphs mark the funnel with lines within which 95% of studies would fall were there no between-study heterogeneity. The choice of the measure of treatment effect and the measure of precision makes a difference to the shape of the plot. Plots of treatment effects against SEs are usually to be preferred, as the funnel will have straight rather than curved sides.[13] However, interpretation of funnel plots can be difficult as there is often an inadequate number of studies. Assessing the causes of funnel plot asymmetry is also difficult because between study heterogeneity; relationships between study quality and sample size; and publication bias, can all cause similar patterns in funnel plots.[14]

7.13 Summary

Multiple logistic regression:
• Report the sample size that the multiple logistic regression model is based on.

- As a minimum give the estimated OR (for the regression coefficient) its confidence interval and associated P-value.
- It is also helpful to give the Hosmer and Lemeshow goodness of fit test value, degrees of freedom and P-value so that the reader can judge whether or not the model adequately fits the data.

Multiple linear regression:
- As a minimum, give the regression coefficient the confidence interval and the P-value.
- It is also helpful to give the R^2 value so that the reader can judge the strength of the relationship.
- It can be helpful to give the SE and the t statistics (ratio of coefficient to SE), and also the residual SD, so that prediction error s can be calculated.

Comparing of two or more groups:
- Each column should represent a different group.
- Each row should represent a different outcome variable.
- The number of observations in each group should be stated. If these differ for different outcome variables (e.g. due to missing values) this should be clear.
- When presenting means, SD and other statistics, consider the precision of the original data. Means should not normally be given to more than one significant figure than the raw data, but SD or SEs may need to be quoted to one extra significant figure.
- For continuous outcomes, the SD should be used to show variability among individuals and the SE of the mean should be used to show the precision of the sample mean. It should be clear which is presented.
- The $\pm$ symbol should not be used to attach the SE or SD to the mean (as in 5.7 $\pm$ 1.6). It is preferable to present these as 5.7 (SE 1.6) or 5.7 (SD 3.6).
- For binary categorical outcomes, report the proportion or percentage of the group who have the outcome of interest along with the numerator and the denominator.
- Percentages should be quoted to no more than 1 decimal for samples of more than 100. With samples of less than 100 the use of decimal places implies unreasonable precision and should be avoided.
- When percentages are contrasted it should be clear whether it is the absolute difference or a relative difference that is being reported. For example, a reduction from 25% to 20% may be expressed as an absolute difference of 5% or a relative difference of 20%.
- Exact P-values (to no more than two significant figures), such as $P = 0.041$ or $P = 0.59$ should be reported. It is not necessary to specify levels of P lower than 0.001 and this can be written as $P < 0.001$ in the table.

- The coverage of the confidence interval (e.g. 90% or 95%) should be clearly stated.
- Confidence intervals should be presented as '−1.4 to 12.8' rather than using the ± symbol or the dash symbol to separate the upper and lower limits.

Randomized controlled trials
- Use the checklist from the CONSORT statement to help with the reporting of the trial.
- Include a flow diagram to describe the flow of patients (and patient numbers) through the trial. Make clear the number of patients randomised and the number of patients with data, available for analysis.
- Summarise the entry or baseline characteristics of the patients in the study groups with suitable summary statistics using an appropriate table. (Data for the study groups should be reported in the columns and the baseline variables by row.)
- Summarise the outcome variables (in rows) for the study groups (in columns) with appropriate summary statistics in a table. Report the estimated treatment effect, and its associated confidence interval (and *P*-value) from the comparison of the outcomes between the study groups.
- Use a forest plot to display the quantitative results of studies included in meta-analyses and systematic reviews. The forest plot can also be used for displaying the results of different outcomes within the same study, provided that they are measured on the same scale.
- Use a funnel plot to detect publication bias in meta-analyses and systematic reviews.

References

1 Morrell CJ, Walters SJ, Dixon S, Collins K, Brereton LML, Peters J, et al. Cost effectiveness of community leg ulcer clinic: randomised controlled trial. *British Medical Journal* 1998;**316**:1487–91.

2 Campbell MJ, Machin D, Walters SJ. *Medical statistics: a textbook for the health sciences*, 4th ed. Chichester: Wiley; 2007.

3 Hosmer DW, Lemeshow S. *Applied logistic regression*, 2nd ed. New York: Wiley; 2000.

4 Thomas KJ, MacPherson H, Thorpe L, Brazier JE, Fitter M, Campbell MJ, et al. Randomised controlled trial of a short course of traditional acupuncture compared with usual care for persistent non-specific low back pain. *British Medical Journal* 2006;**333**:623–6.

5 Bowns IR, Collins K, Walters SJ, McDonagh AJ. Telemedicine in dermatology: a randomised controlled trial. *Health Technology Assessment* 2006;**10**(43):1–58.

6 Simpson AG. A comparison of the ability of cranial ultrasound, neonatal neurological assessment and observation of spontaneous movements to predict outcome in preterm infants University of Sheffield; 2004.

7 Diggle PJ, Heagerty P, Liang K-J, Zeger SL. *Analysis of longitudinal data*, 2nd ed. Oxford: Oxford University Press; 2002.

8 Matthews JNS, Altman DG, Campbell MJ, Royston P. Analysis of serial measurements in medical research. *British Medical Journal* 1990;**300**:230–5.

9 Moher D, Schulz KF, Altman DG, for the CONSORT Group. The CONSORT statement: revised recommendations for improving the quality of reports of parallel group randomised trials. *Lancet* 2001;**357**:1191–4.

10 Altman DG. *Practical statistics for medical research*. London: Chapman & Hall; 1991.

11 Kapoor AS, Kanji H, Buckingham J, Devereaux PJ, McAlister FA. Strength of evidence for perioperative use of statins to reduce cardiovascular risk: systematic review of controlled studies. *British Medical Journal* 2006;**333**:1149–55.

12 Deeks JJ, Everitt B. Forest plot. In: Everitt B, Palmer C, editors. *The encyclopaedic companion to medical statistics*. London: Arnold; 2005.

13 Deeks JJ. Funnel plots. In: Everitt B, Palmer C, editors. *The encyclopaedic companion to medical statistics*. London: Arnold; 2005.

14 Egger M, Davey Smith G, Schnieder M, Minder C. Bias in meta-analysis detected by a simple graphical method. *British Medical Journal* 1997;**315**:629–34.

Appendix

Table A7.1 CONSORT checklist of items to include when reporting a randomised trial[9]

	Item No.	Descriptor
Title and abstract	1	How patients were allocated to interventions.
Introduction		
Background	2	Scientific background and explanation of rationale.
Methods		
Participants	3	Eligibility criteria for participants and the settings and locations where the data were collected.
Interventions	4	Precise details of the interventions intended for each group and how and when they were actually administered.
Objectives	5	Specific objectives and hypotheses.
Outcomes	6	Clearly defined primary and secondary outcome measures and, when applicable, any methods used to enhance the quality of measurements (e.g. multiple observations, training of assessors).
Sample size	7	How sample size was determined and, when applicable, explanation of any interim analyses and stopping rules.
Randomisation		
Sequence generation	8	Method used to generate the random allocation sequence, including details of any restriction (e.g. blocking, stratification).
Allocation concealment	9	Method used to implement the random allocation sequence (e.g. numbered containers or central telephone), clarifying whether the sequence was concealed until interventions were assigned.
Implementation	10	Who generated the allocation sequence, who enrolled participants and who assigned participants to their groups.
Blinding (masking)	11	Whether or not participants, those administering the interventions, and those assessing the outcomes were blinded to group assignment. When relevant, how the success of blinding was evaluated.
Statistical methods	12	Statistical methods used to compare groups for primary outcome(s). Methods for additional analyses, such as subgroup analyses and adjusted analyses.

(Continued)

Table A7.1 (*Continued.*)

	Item No.	Descriptor
Results		
Participant flow	13	Flow of participants through each stage (a diagram is strongly recommended). Specifically, for each group report the numbers of participants randomly assigned, receiving intended treatment, completing the study protocol and analysed for the primary outcome. Describe protocol deviations from study as planned, together with reasons.
Recruitment	14	Dates defining the periods of recruitment and follow-up.
Baseline data	15	Baseline demographic and clinical characteristics of each group.
Numbers analysed	16	Number of participants (denominator) in each group included in each analysis and whether the analysis was by 'intention-to-treat'. State the results in absolute numbers when feasible (e.g. 10/20, not 50%).
Outcomes and estimation	17	For each primary and secondary outcome, a summary of results for each group, and the estimated effect size and its precision (e.g. 95% confidence interval).
Ancillary analyses	18	Address multiplicity by reporting any other analyses performed, including subgroup analyses and adjusted analyses, indicating those pre-specified and those exploratory.
Adverse events	19	Address multiplicity by reporting any other analyses performed, including subgroup analyses and adjusted analyses, indicating those pre-specified and those exploratory.
Discussion		
Interpretation	20	Interpretation of results, taking into account study hypotheses, sources of potential bias or imprecision and the dangers associated with multiplicity of analyses and outcomes.
Generalisability	21	Generalisability (external validity) of the trial findings.
Overall evidence	22	General interpretation of the results in the context of current evidence.

Chapter 8 **Time series plots and survival curves**

8.1 Introduction

This chapter outlines good practice when displaying data that are ordered in time. These data can arise either as a result of the monitoring of a particular event or events across a population over time (time series) or following up individuals over time to measure their time to a particular event (survival analysis). This chapter is not concerned with repeated measures outcome data as they have already been dealt with in Chapter 7.

8.2 Time series plots

A *time series* is a series of observations ordered in time. It differs from the repeated measures data discussed in the previous chapter in two ways:

1 Usually there is only one replication of the data, for example one subject's heart rate monitored over time, or the annual death rates of one country over time. With repeated measures we have more than one subject under consideration.
2 There are many time points. Typically in patient monitoring thousands of points are sampled.

An example of a time series plot is given in Figure 8.1. The data are the number of infant deaths per day in England and Wales over a 7-week period during 1979.[1] The important points to consider when drawing a time series are that time should be on the X-axis (horizontal) and the series of events that are being monitored, the observations, are on the Y-axis (vertical). In addition, adjacent points should be joined by straight lines. If the origin has been omitted this should be made clear, as here, by two diagonal lines on the axis line. Care should be taken when examining published time series plots. They are often used in newspapers and a common trick is not to show the origin, so that a small trend can appear magnified. This is discussed in more detail in Section 2.3.

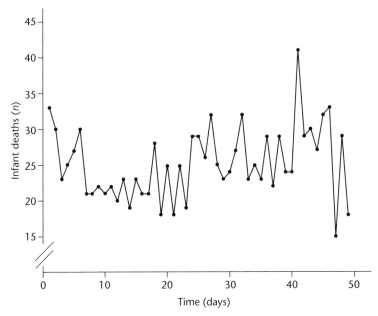

Figure 8.1 Daily infant deaths in England and Wales over a 7-week period during 1979.[1]

8.3 Lowess smoothing plots

Lowess smoothing plots are a useful way of displaying some time series data.[2] They are described in more detail in Section 5.3, where they are applied to continuous data. For time series they are useful for investigating non-linear trends, as demonstrated here. Figure 8.2a shows the number of prescriptions for non-selective serotonin reuptake inhibitors (SSRIs), a type of antidepressant, over a 3.5-year period, from 2002 to 2006 for one general practice in Yorkshire, England (Senior J., Personal Communication, 2006). The scatter plot seems to show a generally increasing trend, with more scatter towards the end. However, fitting a lowess smoothing curve with bandwidth of 50% suggests that in fact the number of prescriptions peaked at around month 30 (Figure 8.2b). This corresponds to the time when national guidelines were published by NICE recommending that SSRIs should be prescribed in preference to non-SSRIs for the treatment of depression. The peak is suggested by the data, and so lowess plots are useful for data exploration, but not for testing hypotheses. Note that as the Y-axis does not begin at the origin (value 0) this has been indicated by two parallel lines.

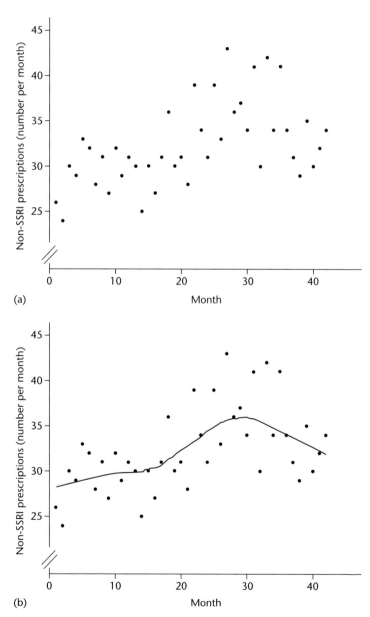

Figure 8.2 Scatterplot and lowess smoothing plot of monthly prescriptions for non-SSRIs antidepressants, for a general practice over 42 months from 2002 to 2006 (Senior J., Personal Communication, 2006): (a) without lowess smoothing plot and (b) with lowess smoothing plot.

8.4 Survival

The major outcome variable in many clinical trials is the time from randomisation and start of treatment to a specified critical event. The length of time from entry to the study to when the critical event occurs is called the survival time. Examples include patient survival time (time from diagnosis to death), length of time that an indwelling cannula remains in situ, or the time a serious burn takes to heal. Even when the final outcome is not an *actual* survival time, the techniques employed with such time-to-event data are conventionally termed 'survival' analysis methods. An important feature of such data is the censored observation, which relates to people who have not suffered an event. Censored observations can happen before the last known follow-up time, if people are lost to follow-up, or they are removed from the 'at risk' dataset for some other reason. Alternatively, they can occur if at the last known follow-up time a number of subjects remain who have not had an event. More details are given in Chapter 10 of Campbell et al.[3]

The conventional plot for survival data is the *Kaplan–Meier survival plot*. This plots the proportion of a group surviving, on the Y-axis, against time, on the X-axis, and allows for censored observations. Figure 8.3 shows a typical

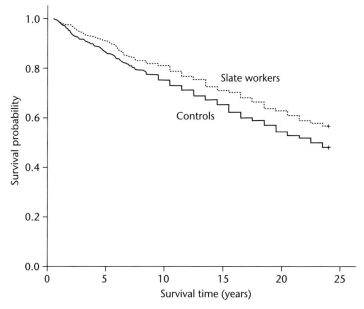

Figure 8.3 Kaplan–Meier survival plot of 25-year follow-up of slate workers ($n = 726$) and controls ($n = 529$).[4]

plot, which displays the survival of 726 slate workers from 1975 to the present day, compared to the survival of 529 controls who were matched by age and smoking habit.[4] Interestingly, the slate workers appear to have better survival than the controls.

However, there are a number of problems with this type of plot. If mortality is low, as it is here, much of the graph is occupied by white space. There is no information about the numbers in each group at particular time points as people die and are censored, the number of people who are at risk at any one time point (number of observations that make up the curves) is reduced. Finally, there is no indication about whether the differences could have arisen by chance.

Particularly when survival is high it is often better to plot mortality (plots going up) rather than survival (plots going down).[5] Though this is not the Kaplan–Meier curve of convention, when mortality is low this can reduce the amount of paper that is blank. Thus Figure 8.4 redraws the earlier data, using the method highlighted by Pocock et al. and addresses the other issues mentioned above. The numbers at risk are included along the horizontal axis and the hazard ratio, together with its corresponding *P*-value has been added to the plot.

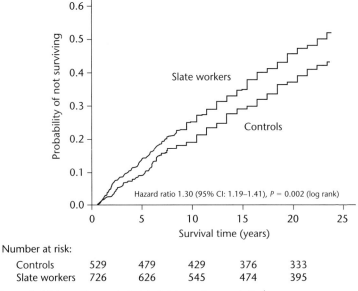

Figure 8.4 Informative survival plot of slate workers mortality.[4]

For some outcomes, where the result is a positive or favourable event, such as a wound or burn healing then it is definitely preferable to have the plots going up, that is, plot the proportion healed. Figure 8.5 gives an example, from the leg ulcer study data used in earlier chapters.[6] All patients began the study with a leg ulcer which was treated either in a specialist clinic or by a district nurse at home. One of the principal outcomes was the time to complete leg ulcer healing. In this example, the vertical axis records the cumulative proportion of patients whose initial leg ulcers healed during the 12-month follow-up period. Figure 8.5 also indicates the censored times as crosses $(+)$ on the lines. This is a useful convention when the amount of data is not too large. Note how the survival curves do not change at these points.

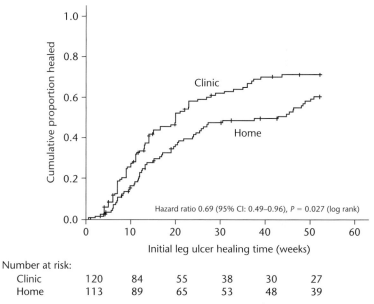

Number at risk:

Clinic	120	84	55	38	30	27
Home	113	89	65	53	48	39

Figure 8.5 Healing times of initial leg ulcers by study group.[6]

Another important problem with conventional survival curves is a tendency to over-interpret the right-hand side of the figure. At this point the curves are based upon fewer and fewer observations because a large proportion of the subjects have already suffered an event, or are censored before that time point. If the longest survival time in each group is associated with a death, then if there are a number of censored data the graph can show an abrupt change. For example the lines in Figure 8.3 would show a sudden drop to zero at the right-hand side if the last person observed had died. It may be sensible only to plot the data until a small percentage (say 10%) of the subjects remain.

Some authors advocate plotting standard errors or confidence intervals on these graphs, but this is not to be recommended, since what is of interest is the contrast between the curves and this is best summarised by a hazard ratio and confidence interval and *P*-value.

Summary

Time series plots:
- Observations should be on the vertical axis and time should be on the horizontal axis.
- Adjacent points should be joined by straight lines.
- Lowess plots can be useful for exploring non-linear trends in time series data.

Survival curves:
- Plot one minus probability of survival on the vertical axis and time on the horizontal axis.
- Clearly label the scales on vertical and horizontal axes.
- Put ticks on the curves at the points where data are censored.
- Show the numbers at risk at suitable time points along the *X*-axis.
- Give some measure of the contrast between curves, such as a hazard ratio and confidence interval or a *P*-value.
- Do not put confidence intervals on individual survival curves.
- Be cautious in interpreting the shape of survival curves. The problems include fewer patients and so poorer estimation at the right-hand end; lack of any pre-specified hypothesis; and lack of power to explore subtleties of curve differences.

References

1 Campbell MJ. Time series regression for counts: an investigation into the relationship between sudden infant death syndrome and environmental temperature. *Journal of the Royal Statistical Society, Series A* 1994;**157**:191–208.
2 Cleveland WS. Robust locally weighted regression and smoothing scatterplots. *Journal of the American Statistical Association* 1979;**74**:829–36.
3 Campbell MJ, Machin D, Walters SJ. *Medical statistics: a textbook for the health sciences*, 4th ed. Chichester: Wiley; 2007.
4 Campbell MJ, Hodges NG, Thomas HF, Paul A, Williams JG. A 24-year cohort study of mortality in slate workers in North Wales. *Journal of Occupational Medicine* 2005;**55**:448–53.

5 Pocock SJ, Clayton TC, Altman DG. Survival plots of time-to-event outcomes in clinical trials: good practice and pitfalls. *Lancet* 2002;**359**:1686–9.

6 Morrell CJ, Walters SJ, Dixon S, Collins K, Brereton LML, Peters J, et al. Cost effectiveness of community leg ulcer clinic: randomised controlled trial. *British Medical Journal* 1998;**316**:1487–91.

Chapter 9 **Displaying results in presentations**

9.1 Introduction

The principle aim of any research presentation or paper is to communicate the results of a study. An important aspect of this is to have an awareness of the intended audience and format available for conveying the relevant information. Whilst the main principle involved when displaying results in either presentations or papers is similar – above all else keep it simple – different formats lend themselves to different types of display, and what is appropriate for a paper or poster may not be appropriate for a presentation. This chapter will focus on how to present information to an audience as part of a seminar or presentation, including how to design good quality, readable slides. These, as much as the person presenting, can make or break a presentation. How to present results in papers has been covered in previous chapters.

When giving an oral presentation to an audience there are several points to be considered. It is important to have an awareness of who the audience are; what information is to be presented and how this information is to be delivered. An integral part of presenting information verbally is having a set of well-designed slides containing information appropriate to the audience. Well-designed slides and good visuals can be enormously useful and greatly enhance a presentation, whilst poorly designed slides with inappropriate visuals can spoil an otherwise informative presentation. Much of this section will be concerned with good slide design, as this is an area that is of fundamental importance when communicating information to an audience: there is little use having good quality tables and charts if the slides themselves are badly designed and difficult to read.

Often presentations, particularly at a conference or seminar have to be given in a limited amount of time and much information has to be conveyed to the audience in that time. Slides should be used to illustrate key points, and should not be read out aloud. As it is possible to elucidate key points verbally in a presentation, there is less need for explanatory text in slides and they should not appear crowded. It is important to think like someone in the audience and to consider what it is that the audience will be seeing and hearing. Charts can be particularly useful as part of a presentation as they can be read quickly, and the key points can be highlighted more easily than if a table were used.

9.2 Graphic design of slides

This section will cover the four basic elements of graphic design as they relate to slide design: text, pictures and graphics, colour, and space. Designing layouts that involve text, pictures, colour and space is not an exact science and there are no hard and fast rules, as what works in one situation will not work in another. Design is about manipulating these four elements. They are all related and it is almost impossible to alter one without it impacting on at least one of the others. For example, the size of the text employed will affect the amount of space available on the slide. However, the following sections will provide some basic guidance to ensure that your slides are legible, understandable and enhance your presentation.

It is important to keep the style of the slides, including the text, colour and any graphic effects consistent throughout a presentation. The choice of font style and graphics can help with the image that you want to portray. The overall look of your slides and the font style and graphics choices are part of the image/impression that you want to convey – be smart in your choices and avoid overly flashy styles. These will distract from your message.

9.3 Text

There is much to consider when thinking about the text used for slides. An initial question concerns the typeface. At their most fundamental, typefaces can be divided into two styles, serif and sans serif typefaces and different ones can be used to create different impressions. Serif typefaces are those with structural details at the end of each stroke. The most commonly used examples are Times New Roman and Garamond (Table 9.1). Whilst Times New Roman is highly legible on paper, it can be difficult for an audience to read on presentation slides and, in general, serif typefaces, particularly the more ornate ones such as Monotype Corsiva, should be avoided for presentations. Sans serif typefaces (from the French 'sans' meaning 'without') do not have flourishes at the end of each letter and common examples include Arial and Verdana (Table 9.1). Sans serif typefaces are easier for an audience to read and should be used for the text on slides. Text is always meant to be read and so

Table 9.1 Examples of common typefaces

Examples of common serif typefaces	Examples of common sans serif typefaces
Times New Roman	Arial
Garamond	Verdana
Book Antiqua	Comic Sans MS

when considering text on slides it is important to bear this principle of legibility in mind Figure 9.1 shows an example of a slide which is overcrowded.

What do we mean when we talk about bivariate data?

- Data where there are two variables
- The two variables can be either categorical, or numerical
- This session we are dealing with continuous bivariate data i.e. both variables are continuous
- We have also looked at categorical bivariate data ...

... categorical bivariate data example from Risk lecture

	Baycol	Other statins
Number who die from rhabdomyolysis	2	1
Number alive or died from other causes	999,998	9,999,999
Total	1,000,000	10,000,000

- There are two binary (categorical) variables
  - Type of stain (Baycol/other)
  - Whether died of rhabdomyolysis or not
- From these data we examined the risk of death from rhabdomyolysis of Baycol compared to other statins

Figure 9.1 Example of over-crowded slide.

No more than two fonts should be used on any slide and text should not take up more than half the visible area. As a good rule of thumb slides should be limited to about six lines of text and no more than six words per line. If this makes it difficult to fit all the points onto a single slide then it is best to break up the points and use more than one slide Figure 9.2 shows how the slide in Figure 9.1 could be split into two slides to improve legibility.

A slide with all the text in capital letters is more difficult to read than a mixture of upper and lower case letters and capitals should only be used for

---

What do we mean when we talk about bivariate data?

- Data where there are two variables
- The two variables can be either
  categorical, or numerical
- This session we are dealing with continuous
  bivariate data i.e. both variables
  are continuous
- We have also looked at categorical
  bivariate data …

(a)

**… categorical bivariate data
example from Risk lecture**

	Baycol	Other statins
Number who die from rhabdomyolysis	2	1
Number alive or died from other causes	999,998	9,999,999
Total	1,000,000	10,000,000

- There are two binary (categorical) variables
  - Type of statin (Baycol / other)
  - Whether died of rhabdomyolysis or not
- From these data we examined the risk of death from
  rhabdomyolysis of Baycol compared to other statins

(b)

Figure 9.2 The same slide split into two separate slides, using a single font type: (a) part 1 of information in Figure 9.1 and (b) part 2 of information in Figure 9.1.

the first character of titles, bullets or names. In general a font size of at least 28 points should be used for the titles and at least 18 points for the main body of the text. As a rough guide if your slide can be read from a distance of about 1 m on a 14 in. computer monitor then it will be legible to an audience when projected (although this will depend upon the size of the room and the size of the screen it is being projected onto).

Text is best highlighted using spacing, italics or colours since underlined or bold text is less easy to read when highlighted. Grouping text can be an effective means of emphasising points and is particularly useful when building up lists

---

And what do the students think?

What did the students find
most useful:

- small group sessions
- lectures and lecture
  notes
- the videos
- first two lectures
- clinical examples
- logical and clear to understand

What did the students find
least useful:

- the group sessions
- the lectures as they are
  too hard
- the videos
- the early sessions
- clinical scenarios
- too much stats

Figure 9.3 Use of bullet points to emphasise key points.

of opposing views, although it can make the slide layout more complex. Figure 9.3 illustrates this using some data taken from a survey of medical students asking them about the medical statistics teaching that they had received. As part of this teaching they were asked what they had found most and least useful about the teaching. On the left-hand side are what they had found most useful and on the right-hand side what they had found least useful. In this slide the presenter is able to contrast how similar the two lists are – whilst some students found the small group useful, others did not, and whilst some students wanted more mathematics, others found the level already too difficult.

The lists in Figure 9.3 use bullet points to emphasise key points. Bulleted lists can be an effective way of guiding an audience through the main points of a slide, particularly when used in combination with the animation feature so that each point appears in order as and when required. In keeping with the recommended number of lines, it is best to have no more than six bullet points on a slide, have them appear one at a time without special effects and then have them 'grey out' as the next one appears. This will give greater control of pace. There are a great many different animation effects that can be used with bulleted lists, but the simplest is the best, otherwise a presentation can appear rather gimmicky and detract from the message being presented.

9.4 Pictures/graphics: including the use of graphics and clip art

With pictures, clip art and graphics animations it is easy to get carried away with 'gee-whiz' effects. However, it is worth resisting the temptation as much as possible, to ensure that the audience remain focussed on you and your message. Use only those that are absolutely integral to the presentation as anything else will look flashy and as stated previously will detract from the information being presented. Having said this, provided they are relevant and suit the subject material they can be useful for livening up an otherwise dull presentation, particularly if the subject matter is rather dry. By using animations sparingly they will have a greater impact when you do use them. One final note on animation effects is the use of slide transitions. These are the effects that are applied to slides as the presentation moves from one slide to the next. Although many different ones exist, as with other advice throughout this chapter, keep it simple. The more elaborate a transition effect, the more it will detract from a serious presentation.

9.5 Colour

The appropriate use of colour can greatly enhance a presentation, but as with all other aspects of slide design there are a few guidelines that can improve its use. The two most important areas where colour can be used are with the text and with the background. When projected onto a screen, light coloured text against a dark background (either as a solid colour or shaded gradient) works best.

Colour can be used to highlight text within a slide but care should be taken to not get carried away with lots of different colours. No more than three colours should be used on a single slide. It is important to consider the combination of colours to be used, as some colours work well together whilst others do not. Briefly, there are three primary colours, red, blue and yellow and these, together with black and white can be used to form any other colour. When two of the primary colours are mixed together they form the secondary colours, orange (red and yellow), purple (blue and red) and green (blue and yellow). These colours can then be arranged in a circle to form a colour wheel as in Figure 9.4. Colours that are opposite each other on the colour wheel will contrast with each other (complementary colours), whilst those that are close will harmonise with each other. A more complex colour wheel can be found at http://www.shef.ac.uk/scharr/sections/hsr/statistics/staff/freeman.html.

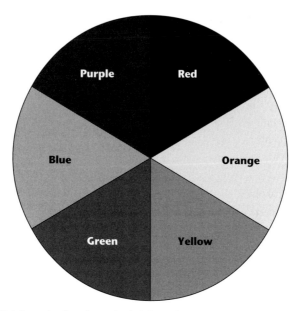

Figure 9.4 Example of a colour wheel. Colours close to each other will harmonise, whilst those opposite each other will contrast.

In using colour, it is worth remembering that different colours have different cultural connotations and some colour combinations can be especially difficult for people with particular conditions such as dyslexia or colour blindness to read. Consider for example the effect of using both red and green to highlight contrasting points in the text – this will be virtually indistinguishable for individuals with colour blindness.

9.6 Space

Space is as important as the other elements detailed above and it is essential not to overcrowd slides as they will look busy and be difficult to read. Space can be used to break up text and to highlight specific points. If there is a lot of text on a slide, consider breaking it up and creating two slides, as in Figure 9.2. This is also true of subheadings as these can make a slide look crowded. These are best avoided and it is better to break major points into separate slides rather than have subheadings. As stated in the section on text, as a general guide there should be no more than six lines of text per slide and six words per line.

9.7 Summary slides

Always include an outline slide at the beginning of the presentation and a conclusion slide at the end. These should include 3–5 summary points that focus on the main points. The first slide should outline what the talk is about and guide the audience through the forthcoming presentation whilst the summary slide should emphasise the 'take home' message and focus on the final impression that you want to convey. It is hard to over-emphasise the main points as it is important for your audience to be sure of what the talk is about.

9.8 Conclusion

Much of this chapter has concentrated on the graphic design of slides. It should be noted that although getting the 'look' of the presentation is important, this should not be at the expense of the content. Graphic design is as much about 'who' and 'why' as about 'how'. Design is often thought of as being about how to make something look attractive, but before thinking about how something should look it is important to be sure that you say the right thing to the right people in the right way: always keep in mind your target audience and desired aims.

Summary

- Keep slides simple.
- Text is meant to be read. Ensure that your slides are legible.
- For slides use light text on a dark background.
- Keep information layout, colours, patterns, text styles, and transitions and build effects consistent for all slides in a presentation.
- Maximum of six lines per slide and six words per line.
- Use graphics and animation effects sparingly.
- San serif fonts such as Arial are the more legible for slides.
- Use a minimum font size of 28 points for titles and 18 points for the body of text.

Index

DATE DUE